FLEXIBLE BODIES

FLEXIBLE BODIES

TRACKING IMMUNITY IN AMERICAN CULTURE—FROM THE DAYS OF POLIO TO THE AGE OF AIDS

EMILY MARTIN

BEACON PRESS

Boston

Beacon Press
25 Beacon Street
Boston, Massachusetts 02108-2892

Beacon Press books
are published under the auspices of
the Unitarian Universalist Association of Congregations.

Library of Congress Cataloging-in-Publication Data

Martin, Emily.
    Flexible bodies: tracking immunity in American culture —
from the days of polio to the age of AIDS / Emily Martin.
        p.   cm.
    Includes bibliographical references and index.
    ISBN 0-8070-4626-4 (cloth)
    ISBN 0-8070-4627-2 (paper)
    1. Medical anthropology—United States.   2. Immunity—Social
aspects.   3. Immune system—Social aspects.   4. Americans—Health
and hygiene.   I. Title.
GN296.5.U6M37   1994
306.4'61—dc20   93-39065

99 98 97 96   8 7 6 5 4 3

Text design by Ruth Kolbert

For Richard

*Indeed, people don't just become ill out of the blue. For the whole
of a body to be affected, its equilibrium must have already been
disrupted. That's true for all illnesses. It's painfully obvious for
illnesses said to be of the immune system. But all illnesses are, in fact,
since being ill comes down to being unable to distance oneself from
pathogenic agents. So why do we have this proliferation of terminal
illnesses at a period of civilization as developed as ours? My
hypothesis is that it's this very civilization that continuously
submits our minds and bodies to stresses and strains and thus
gradually destroys our immune systems. I'm surprised doctors
aren't saying this.*
LUCE IRIGARAY, *Je, Tu, Nous: Toward a Culture of Difference*

*There may be something of fundamental significance in the fact that
a well-known credit card was advertised as "your flexible friend."*
ROGER PAIN, *"Protein Dynamics: A Case of a Flexible Friend"*

Tertio agemus de corporibus flexibilibus.
LEONHARD EULER, *Mechanica*

CONTENTS

ILLUSTRATIONS

PREFACE

In 1951, my brother had polio during an epidemic and died at the age of two when I was seven. I can recall vividly my fear of germs in general, the injunctions against being in crowds or swimming pools or having unwashed hands. I recall how I was allowed to see my paralyzed brother only from outside, through the closed window of his hospital ward, for fear of his contagion. I recall how my family was quarantined by means of an order from the Department of Public Health for fear of our contagion.

What has happened since those times to make public health recommendations for management of the AIDS epidemic today so different? I have recently been spending time daily as a volunteer in very close proximity to people with advanced cases of AIDS. To be sure, HIV's route of transmission, so very different from polio's, makes fear of simple proximity unnecessary. But it was a striking contrast to me that as for all the other "opportunistic" diseases my companions with HIV/AIDS had — such as tuberculosis, herpes, or toxoplasmosis — I believed I did not have to worry. In my training to be a volunteer, I had often been told that only those with impaired immune systems would be susceptible. The germs themselves posed no threat as long as my immune system was strong. How had this change come about? In this book, my concern is how our taken-for-grantedness about the body is generated. How is it different from the taken-for-grantedness of only twenty or thirty years ago? And is this change in what is taken for granted about health related to other dramatic changes in the United States?

It is incontrovertible that, in the course of approximately the last two decades, the configuration and organization of many parts of the social order in the United States have been undergoing dramatic and fundamental shifts. Some of these shifts can be shown to result from large-scale economic changes, such as the move to a global, international economic market. Some are occurring in a great variety of different domains, in varying degrees, and sometimes with little, if any, demonstrable casual relation to each other. The shifts that especially concern me in this book relate to the questions of what "health" is, what it includes, what a body is made up of, what a person is made up of, what makes a healthy work organization, what disease is, and how the terms in which people come to understand themselves yield particular answers to questions like these.

To learn the answers to the questions I have posed, I have relied heavily on extended, informal interviews with more than two hundred people in many walks of life. Simultaneously, to learn something about knowledge produced in the science of biology, I began participant-observation in a research lab in immunology in which I was able to attend classes, lab meetings, journal clubs (for the discussion of current articles), lectures, and parties. Later, I was taught to perform Western blots, a technical procedure used in the lab (routine for them, fabulously complex for me), and participated in carrying out part of a series of experiments.

I also started to work as a volunteer in one of Baltimore's main AIDS service organizations, HERO. Although I had no idea at the start whether it was possible to do research as a volunteer, research and volunteer working seeming potentially incompatible, I could not think how else to proceed. I was not a member of the gay and lesbian community in Baltimore, and I had not had to deal directly with HIV-related issues in my life. But, in the tradition of fieldworking anthropologists in other parts of the world, it did seem possible, if I put my body there as well as my eyes and mouth, so to speak, that I could learn at least something about the experiences being produced by HIV/AIDS. From the first moment at HERO and in all other contexts in which I worked as a volunteer, I told everyone that I was an anthropologist doing a research project on health in the United States. This sometimes created complications, but the general reaction was, "Oh, that's interesting; now when can you show up to work?"

I was interviewed for and accepted into HERO's "buddy" training program, trained to be a buddy, and immediately started work at a residential home for HIV+ people. Over the next three years, I was a primary buddy to three HIV+ individuals and interacted less intensely with many others. As stipulated by HERO, I attended a biweekly support group for buddies. Later, I was trained to lead and undertook to co-lead a buddy support group.

During the first year of the project, I also joined ACT UP/BALTO, again in the double capacity of anthropologist/volunteer. Experiences with ACT UP allowed me to see the politics of AIDS from a particular point of view. One of ACT UP's most powerful techniques is to make its presence felt dramatically at a public event. When you are at an event as an ACT UP member, blowing a shrieking horn, holding an effigy of the governor, or dramatically falling "dead" on the ground, there is no hiding in the background. At the first demonstration I attended, to protest the inaction of Governor's AIDS Commission, a terrific thunderstorm with violent lightning burst on us as we marched in front of the building where the commission was meeting. The next day, a newspaper published a photograph of the group of us, with me in the middle looking up bewildered and fearful at the exploding sky. In this case I was reacting to the storm, but more often I felt fearful and bewildered because of the potential for violence, both verbal and physical, entailed in these confrontations. As in the cases of working in the lab and being a buddy for people who were suffering from AIDS, I felt an imperative to place myself bodily in these contexts, to feel viscerally the threats and dangers as well as the delights of working and organizing to fight this major epidemic in the late twentieth century.

What might be called *visceral learning* has long been a part of fieldwork in the anthropological sense and is often what sets anthropological work off from that of other disciplines. Maurice Bloch believes that most of what anthropologists learn is gained precisely through these kinds of nonlinguistic, felt experiences, not through the answers to verbal questions put directly to people (Bloch 1991). Surely we depend on both kinds of learning, and surely it is the mutual interplay between them both that is the most informative aspect of ethnography. Accordingly, in all the contexts in which I participated as a volunteer, I also interviewed as many people as possible.

As is usually the case for anthropologists, moving among such places was complex: I was never simply inside or simply outside any one group. One day I heard about the results of the latest AZT trials in a meeting of ACT UP, while planning a demonstration to cruelly embarrass the Mayor's AIDS Commission. The next day I heard about the same trials at immunology grand rounds, where I could have asked doctors a question that related directly to the well-being of my current buddy. The following day, while playing my assigned role in the "zap" against the Mayor's Commission (which seemed to have the desired embarrassing effect), I faced the reproachful look of the member of the mayor's staff who had gone far out of the way to help me gain access to ordinarily confidential materials concerning Baltimore's efforts to restructure its conceptions and practices concerning health, public education, and worker training.

My fieldwork has made clear to me that the categories of social analysis that we once found so useful to describe our lives — gender, race, class, work, home, family, community, state and nation, science and religion — are no longer sufficient to describe, let alone analyze, the phenomena of the contemporary metropolis: the couple who, having been laid off their "lifetime" jobs at IBM, now run a business out of their home using a computer and a fax machine; the young woman who works at a trendy restaurant in the Inner Harbor but has to sleep under a bridge at night; the automobile line worker who gives an invited talk at a national conference on work redesign about the engineering innovations that his team has invented in his Japanese-owned company; the schoolteacher who abandons all his medicines and goes to live near the church community in which he has been restored to health after being fully symptomatic with AIDS for several years; the M.D. who says "we know so little about the body" and pursues homeopathic remedies for her child's recurring infections; the African-American manager of human resources who organizes "diversity training" for the state department of agriculture. These people, or people equally as complicated, walk the pages of the book that follows. Some different means of description must be found, for they have surely already broken the terms of our old categories, and pushing their lives back into those categories will not advance our understanding. Since, under the kinds of wrenching change that I observed during the research, the very borders of the sociological entities such as work, family, community, and science are often in flux, it did not seem advisable to begin with them as the units of analysis.

A theme that runs through the book is this: that what goes to make up a person in these times is being reconfigured. Is the traditional "person" (sometimes called the *subject*) dissolving? In reference to the increasingly common computerized calculation of risk factors for the hazards of disease among populations, Paul Rabinow notes that "individuals sharing certain traits or sets of traits can be grouped together in a way that not only decontextualizes them from their social environment but also is nonsubjective in a double sense: it is objectively arrived at, and does not apply to, a subject in anything like the older sense of the word (that is, the suffering, meaningfully situated integrator of social, historical, and bodily experiences)" (1992a:243). The chapters that follow show, from a variety of angles, what it is like to be such a "subject" whose accustomed terms of experience are undergoing some spectacular shifts.

Many of these shifts, as we will see, involve the emergence of the immune system as a field in terms of which all manner of questions and definitions about health are given meaning and measured. In our fieldwork, no matter how far away from immunology labs and HIV/AIDS contexts we went, even into the training sessions of Fortune 500 corporations, we found people actively using the immune system to organize and comprehend their lives.

Partly in connection with this emergence of the immune system, one of our new taken-for-granted virtues for persons and their bodies has come to be "flexibility." Arising as a trait to be cherished and cultivated, from corporations and city governments to credit cards and shoes, flexibility is an object of desire for nearly everyone's personality, body, and organization. Flexibility has also become a powerful commodity, something scarce and highly valued, that can be used to discriminate against some people.

We are at a moment when new sources of power are emerging in American culture. Understanding better the links between science and society may help us avoid one of the bleakest potential consequences of these new models of the ideal flexible body — that, yet again, certain categories of people (women, people of color) will be found wanting. Certain social groups may be seen as having rigid or unresponsive selves and bodies, making them relatively unfit for the kind of society we seem now to desire. Another possible consequence — no less bleak — is that the old categories of hierarchical discrimination will be reshuffled in fundamental ways. A conception of a new elite may be forged that finds the desirable qualities of flexibility and adaptability to change in certain superior individuals of *any* ethnic, racial, gender, sexual identity, or age group in the nation. The "currency" in which these desirable qualities will be figured is health, especially the health of one's immune system. What will be forged is a conception of "fitness" in which, just as surely as in nineteenth-century social Darwinism (although the terms and mechanisms may differ), some will survive and some will not.

ACKNOWLEDGMENTS

The circle of helpers and supporters who enabled me to write this book is very wide. Occupying the largest part of the ring, and enabling everything else, were the graduate students who, as part of their graduate programs in anthropology at Johns Hopkins, acted as field-workers on this project. There is no way adequately to encompass in words the gratitude I feel for the hard work, original insights, long patience, steady commitment, and skillful ethnography of Bjorn Claeson, Laury Oaks, Wendy Richardson, Monica Schoch-Spana, and Karen-Sue Taussig. During each of the three years of the project, three of them were involved as field-workers.

In my mind's eye, I remember each of these students at a particular moment that epitomizes for me his or her unique contribution. I remember Bjorn's earnest seriousness while watching a science film with a group of high school students studying for their high school equivalency degree and his wide-eyed appreciation as the students revealed and demolished the metaphoric structure of the film. I remember Laury's sage counsel, and giggles, as we discussed what we should wear to a total quality management seminar on being a "successful woman." I remember Wendy's gentle sensitivity as we attended meetings of a polio support group and tried, without giving offense, to interview some of its members. I remember Monica's unaffected interest and social grace as we attended a seminar designed to teach new owners of low-income houses how to plunge a toilet, change a furnace filter, and free a stuck garbage disposal. I remember Karen-Sue's courage, and hilarity, as we made our way through a day on a high ropes course for the training of corporate employees, leaping off poles, climbing towers, and, finally, her pluck as she was chosen as the member of our small group who would be hoisted by rope over a make-believe "acid lake" in a problem-solving exercise.

During the last year of research, Ariane van der Straten joined the group. With her special background — a Ph.D. in molecular biology — and her new career plans — to begin graduate school in anthropology or public health — she was able to conduct some of the research in medical and scientific settings very effectively. That year, Anne Lorimer, a graduate student in the Department of Anthropology at the University of Chicago, also joined the group, at a distance, by working through many boxes of interviews on health in the archives of the National Opinion Research Center (NORC) in Chicago.

This collaboration, entailing full financial support for the students, was enabled by generous funding from the Spencer Foundation and would in no way have been possible without it. Of course, the research itself, as well as the conclusions reached in this book, are solely my responsibility. At the end of the three years, I enjoyed a year of writing in the delightfully serene environment of the Institute for Advanced Study, where I was a Mellon fellow. I am grateful to the faculty of the School of Social Sciences at the institute and the Andrew W. Mellon Foundation for enabling my stay.

Portions of earlier versions of parts of the book, now in a very different form, were published in the *Medical Anthropology Quarterly* (December 1990), in *Culture, Medicine and Psychiatry* (1993), and in the *American Ethnologist* (February 1992). I thank these publications, the American Anthropological Association, and Kluwer Academic Publishers for permission to reprint here. Parts of the book were discussed in seminars or presented in lectures at various universities and academic settings, including the University of Chicago, the University of Kentucky, the University of Manchester, the University of Essex, the Wellcome Institute for the History of Medicine, the London School of Economics, the School for Oriental and African Studies, Rennselear Polytechnic Institute, the Women's Studies Seminar at Johns Hopkins University, the Society for Cultural Anthropology, the Canadian Anthropological Society, the Association of Social Anthropologists of the British Commonwealth, the Social Science Research Council conference on "Immunization and Culture," the Wenner-Gren conference on "The Politics of Reproduction," and the conference on "Sex/Gender in Technoscience Worlds" at the University of Melbourne. I feel very grateful for the enormous amount of stimulating discussion from which I benefited on these occasions.

To those who helped us negotiate the numerous settings in which the research was conducted — in research labs, clinics, support groups, nursing homes, neighborhoods, and workplaces — I thank you all for taking a risk with us, for believing in the worth of the project even when we had trouble making clear what its results would be. In the book, I use pseudonyms for all who are quoted in interviews, but, for their invaluable help in facilitating our initial access to field settings, I would like to thank by name Jackie Adams, Patrick Bova, Michael Edidin, Elizabeth Fee, Kathleen Galloway, Jasper Hunt, Jimmy Jones, Joyce Kramer, Paul Lewis, Doris McElroy, David Neumann, Noel Rose, Terry Ryder, Liza Solomon, John Stuban, Lee Tawney, and David Vlahof. Marshall Sahlins provided essential material support by lending space in his office for Anne Lorimer to store and read NORC interviews. My sister, Katrina Prull, introduced me to the existence of antivaccination sentiment in the United States and told me how to get access to the relevant materials.

For the things I learned while working together on common tasks, I want to thank, with affection, Barbara Greene and Laura Gregorzak, my "co-buddies," and Greg Allen and David Neumann, my mentors in the Western blot. My appreciation also goes to every person who agreed to talk to us, either in an interview or more informally. While some of you said that our questions made you "feel important," and others said that they made you "feel like a dummy," I am indebted to you all.

Numerous colleagues and friends played a significant role during the research and writing of this book, bolstering my spirits, reacting to my ideas, or generally encouraging me to carry on: Bill Arney, Sarah Begus, Lisa Croll, Barbara Duden, Susan Harding, Ruth Hubbard, Ludmilla Jordanova, Henrietta Moore, Mary Poovey, Lorna Rhodes, Erica Schoenberger, Jane Sewell, Sharon Stephens, Marilyn Strathern, and Margery Wolf. Susan Harding, Laury Oaks, Mary Poovey, Karen-Sue Taussig, Ariane van der Straten, and the members of the Cyborg Anthropology Seminar at the School of American Research gave me detailed commentary on part or all of the manuscript in its nearly final form. I thank you all deeply, but you are not, of course, responsible for any errors that remain.

All my colleagues in the Department of Anthropology at Johns Hopkins were, as they have always been, supportive friends as well as stimulating intellectual companions: Gillian Feeley-Harnik, Ashraf Ghani, Niloofar Haeri, Sidney Mintz, Rolph Trouillot, and Katherine Verdery. My temporary colleagues during my year at the Institute for Advanced Study had a special role to play in the writing of this book because the theme for the year was the social study of science. I especially thank Clifford Geertz for clarifying my sense that the social study of science could gain by going beyond the laboratory, Freeman Dyson for introducing me to Richard Preston, and Shawn Marmon and Doris Kaufmann for neighborly company and rousing conversations in the "girls' dorm."

As always in a study of this kind, some of the most important labor takes place in offices and libraries outside the field settings proper. I want to thank the two people who did the vast majority of transcribing the over two hundred taped interviews on which the study is based: Patricia Masselink and Jackie Nguyen. Both of them were meticulously careful, endlessly patient, and willing to endure the discomfort to eyes, ears, back, neck, arms, and head that so frequently accompanies extended work at a video terminal. Susan Gershman, Josh Coleman, and Bret McCabe were undergraduates who gave an enormous amount of energy and care to transcribing tapes, finding library materials, and photocopying. As in the past, I was immensely aided in gathering far-flung research materials by the efficient and speedy services of the Inter-Library Loan Department and the Eisenhower Express at Eisenhower Library; I also appreciate the help of Marsha Tucker in the Historical Studies/Social Science Library of the Institute for Advanced Study.

For her sound editorial advice, consistent support, and calm in the face of my occasional panic, I thank Lauren Bryant at Beacon Press. For his outstanding copyediting, I thank Joseph Brown. For shoring up my psychic infrastructure, I thank Ellen McDaniel and Joan Bielefeld.

Finally, I come to the home team. Every member of my immediate family was a participant in this research and made an inestimable contribution to it. In this context, I can mention only a few of the ways in which they were involved. Ariel, at age nine, was my field assistant at the Experiential Education Association meeting in Lake Junaleska, N.C. She bravely went off by herself with a bunch of kids she had never met, to join the "Kidference" that paralleled the main conference, where, for the first time, she rode a mountain bike that was too big for her, down roads that were too narrow, in hopes of being able to tell me about experiential education for children. She was a source of joy for my buddies, who did not often have visits from young children at the end of their illnesses, and she did an excellent job arranging many baskets of fruit and vases of flowers for them. Jenny, at age sixteen, was my moral support during the painful memorial service for my first buddy, Mark. Had she not been with me, I would not have tried as hard as I did to reach the other volunteers who had not been told about the service, and I do not know whether I would have been able to stand up and speak to the group about Mark at all. She also helped me keep my sanity and perspective during meetings of a subgroup of ACT UP devoted to getting Mr. Condom (a six-foot-high body mask in the shape of a condom wearing a cheerful face) into the hallways of some Baltimore high schools.

My husband, Richard, was my constant tutor in the ways of physiology and immunology. He never tired of translating arcane biological terminology and spelling out the implications of different theoretical starting points. He took me along to more than one workshop or conference on immunology to which I did not really have an invitation, and he introduced me to lots of scientists. He was a good friend to my buddy Mark, and he smoothed away my (and our childrens') fears of contracting HIV infection from all the contact we were having with extremely sick people. Only much later did I find out he was scared himself. In his life and work, he has set me a model to emulate of doing research that grapples with the most serious and compelling human problems that exist. This book is for him.

$\mathscr{P}$ART
ONE

INTRODUCTION: PROBLEMS AND METHODS

Managers who recognise the nature of bounded instability will also design actions to deal with the open-ended nature of change over the long term. They will recognise that open-ended change removes all the conditions required for the practice of the planning and ideological modes of control and development. They will therefore abandon all attempts at long-term planning and envisioning as a comprehensive means of developing the business over the long term. They will rely instead on complex learning in groups to produce emergent intention, strategy, culture and business philosophy. They will accept the inevitable unpredictability and irregularity of the innovative, the creative and the new.

RALPH STACEY, *Managing Chaos*

THE ENCYCLOPEDIA BRITANNICA PUBLISHES AN ANNUAL VOLUME, called *The Great Ideas Today,* that is meant to supplement and update the more than fifty-volume *The Great Books of the Western World.* In *The Great Ideas Today, 1991,* the lead article was titled "The Biology of Immune Responses." Written by Michael Edidin, a colleague of mine at Johns Hopkins, it is one of only two pieces in the volume that deal with a scientific topic: it sits uneasily among the other articles about modern dance, multiculturalism, music as a liberal art, theology, and so on. Edidin (1991:2) begins his article with this passage:

> The fortress of Acre ('Akko) rises out of the Mediterranean Sea on the coast of Israel. It is an elaborate and beautiful structure; its great stone seawalls are topped with towers, and its courts connect by arched tunnels. The fortress is a history of the region. Its oldest parts, now half-hidden by sea or earth, were built by the Crusaders, and it was elaborated, extended, and modernized by the Turks. Its structure and complexity remind the immunologist of another great complex that protects against invasion — the complex of organs, cells, and molecules that functions as our immune system.

My recent research focuses on the history of the meaning of Edidin's topic: the immune system. When I began the research, in

1989, it was an open question for me whether anyone outside an immunology lab or a specialized clinic would know or care anything about something called *the immune system*. By the time Edidin's article was published in 1991, I felt that I was beginning to have some grasp of the processes that led the Britannica editors to regard the immune system as one of "the great ideas today."

Understanding the genealogy of the immune system, a task too large to be completed in any single book, led me to place the recent eminence of the immune system in the context of how our notions about health, the body, and disease have changed since the 1940s and 1950s. My intent in juxtaposing the present and the recent past is to "defamiliarize present practices and categories, to make them seem less self-evident and necessary" (Sawicki 1991:101), to describe at least some of the "connections, encounters, supports, blockages, plays of forces, strategies and so on which at a given moment establish what subsequently counts as being self-evident, universal and necessary" (Foucault 1991:76).

I imagined that our understanding of the immune system must somehow involve developments in biological science and their dissemination to the public. But I had reason to doubt how salient the affairs of scientific investigation would be outside science, especially since the idea of the immune system as a system of interacting parts, an "all encompassing framework," has existed in science only since the 1970s (Moulin 1989:293). It is commonly asserted by many philosophers, historians, sociologists, and anthropologists that natural science occupies a domain separate from the rest of daily social life. In part this separation is understood as a result of the growing professionalization and secularization of science: whereas in the past most people thought that moral, social, and political issues ought to be brought to bear on how nature was understood, in the present most people think that good and proper science should be carried on autonomously, completely separate from such issues (Shapin 1982:175).

In part the autonomy we are willing to attribute to contemporary science is maintained by scientists themselves, who assert in various ways that "the layman and the non-specialist are posited in the natural sciences as ones whose interpretation of, and opinion about, the works of science *ought* not intrude into the relevant discussions at all. Their views are culturally fixed as in principle irrational, or at least irrelevant" (Markus 1987:22). This maintenance of strict boundaries around who can legitimately speak about scientific knowledge has consequences for scientists as well as the rest of us: drastically negative sanctions await scientists who appeal to the general public for an opinion about their research before seeking certification by professional peers.

The overall picture assumed in the present day is that knowledge of the natural world is produced by scientists doing proper science. This knowledge is concentrated in its purest form in the scientists who produce it; then, to a limited extent, it filters out or trickles down to other professional groups or the general public. In the filtering or trickling process, scientific knowledge, it is often feared, becomes distorted, partial, and misleading. It is this picture that lends energy to the recent outcry over the lack of "science literacy" among people in the United States. People fail to answer correctly many questions on tests devised by scientists to measure their quotient of scientific knowledge. One question from a newspaper quiz is the following.

> The blueprint for every form of life is contained in
> a. The National Institutes of Health near Washington, D.C.
> b. DNA molecules
> c. Proteins and carbohydrates
> d. Viruses. (Hazen and Trefil 1991:26)

Those people who do not know the correct answer (or think that it might be open to debate!) are exhorted to take remedial action by reading special books written by scientists to encapsulate in simple terms the knowledge that science has produced about the world, such as *Science Matters* (Hazen and Trefil 1991b) or *The New York Times Book of Science Literacy* (Flaste 1991).

But this common picture is only one way to sketch the relationship between science and the public. When observers pay careful attention to how people conduct their daily lives, they find the very same people who might well fail school tests in math, for example, successfully using sophisticated mathematical calculations and estimations (Lave 1988:145–69; Douglas 1985:32–33). In anthropologist Jean Lave's study, even though supermarket shoppers "had not the slightest idea that they were extraordinarily efficacious at arithmetic problem solving," they did not make many errors in the final outcome of their price calculations. Shoppers correctly calculated the best buy 90 percent of the time. In contrast, in figuring comparable problems in a test setting, the same people averaged only 57 percent correct (Lave 1986:92, 104).

Complicating the picture further, when sociological observers began to enter the places where scientific knowledge is produced, the laboratory, they found many practices that seemed to share more with daily life outside the lab than with the strict edicts governing knowledge in science, such as universality, objectivity, or reproducibility. Measurement of the presence or absence of a substance might be based on a very unclear sign, blurry and indistinct, whose reading depended on a local consensus. Techniques might be developed in local settings and depend on local materials and practices (Knorr-Cetina 1981, 1983). When experiments are replicated, the process or entity previously "discovered" might turn out not to be there at all (Latour and Woolgar 1986). The establishment of findings in the laboratory as facts accepted by the wider scientific community might turn out to be in large part a social process, a process of gaining credibility from a group of peers through means given legitimacy in the scientific community: scholarly publication, successful grant application, laboratory work, more publication, and so on (Latour and Woolgar 1986; Latour 1987).

As observers of science in the laboratory followed its products into the wider society, they found that essentially social and political factors turned out to play the dominant role in whether and how these products continued to exist outside the laboratory. Sometimes, as in the case of Pasteur's discoveries about anthrax, some of the conditions of the laboratory, such as measurement, timing, disinfecting, recording, etc., had to be imposed on the farms in which trials of the efficacy of the method were carried out. The conditions of the laboratory had to be extended into the world outside it (Latour 1983, 1988).

For all that we have learned from the rich lode that laboratory studies have mined, there is one area that they leave relatively untouched. These studies share something of the perspective of scientists themselves about the primacy and power of the knowledge that they are producing. Scientists, albeit with procedures that have turned out to be different from those employed in their own idealized pictures, are always the active agents in these scenarios: they translate, read, write, mobilize, impose, convince. They may succeed or fail at imposing their knowledge on the world outside science or even on their own colleagues, but they are always pictured as active agents attempting to change an essentially passive world. Pasteur has to mobilize the farmers, but the farmers are not seen as exerting influence on the scientists.[1]

Corrective work is now being done that is beginning to change this picture, work that is largely ethnographic research conducted by anthropologists. Working with a conviction that what scientists do can be seen as embedded within a complex cultural world with historical depth, anthropologists have begun to reveal the intricacies of describing the work of scientists in the context of a world that is not assumed to be passive (Hess 1992). We can now understand the significance of the man who used legal restraints to force scientists to include him in the profits yielded by a product of his cells. The finding in the case was motivated in part by very old ideas in Western culture about the inviolability of the human body — his cells were *his* no matter how they had been enhanced by scientific techniques (Rabinow 1992b). We can also understand the complex religious, moral, economic, and social grounds on which families accept or reject the use of genetic knowledge about a growing fetus (Rapp 1988). The same chromosomal "defect" could be interpreted as an acceptable variation within the norm by a working-class family concerned more about physical integrity than mental acuity or as an unacceptable deformity by an upper-middle-class family far more concerned about their children scaling the heights of intelligence charts than about putting up with a minor physical abnormality.

In this book, I assume as a starting point that seeing science as an active agent in a culture that passively acquiesces does not provide an adequately complex view of how scientific knowledge operates in a social world. I deliberately cross back and forth across the borders between the institutions in which scientists produce knowledge (an immunology research laboratory, clinical settings) and the wider society (neighborhoods, places of work). (One of my colleagues in science studies was disturbed by this departure from the laboratory as the only site of research and asked me, "Don't you know how to stay put!?") To avoid the idealized picture of science, which its practitioners would like to believe, that knowledge is produced inside and flows out, I would like to consider an alternative series of guiding metaphors altogether.

Toward this end, I have found it useful to borrow the image of culture as an old city surrounded by modern suburbs, an image developed by Clifford Geertz from an analogy that Wittgenstein used to describe language: "a maze of little streets and squares, of old and new houses,

and of houses with additions from various periods; and this surrounded by a multitude of new boroughs with straight regular streets
and uniform houses" (Wittgenstein 1953:8). Geertz extends this image
to culture: "We can say that anthropologists have traditionally taken the
old city for their province, wandering about its haphazard alleys trying
to work up some rough sort of map of it, and have only lately begun to
wonder how the suburbs, which seem to be crowding in more closely
all the time, got built, what connection they have to the old city . . . and
what life in such symmetrical places could possibly be like." In this
image, the sciences are taken to be "squared off and straightened out
systems of thought and action" (Geertz 1983a:73–74) that form the
modern, suburban sections of the city.

    This image has the merit of suggesting that culture can simultane-
ously involve structures built in different time periods and that the
inhabitants of those structures might be able to move about the landscape. To increase its usefulness for my analysis, I need to add a few
elements: at a minimum, electronic media for transporting images,
words, and ideas between the old city, the new suburbs, the rest of the
country, and the world. This has the potential of upsetting the way in
which we might imagine inhabitants in various parts of the city to be
linked to processes impelling change. For example, a scientist who
works (and because of her devotion practically lives) in the metaphoric
"modern suburbs" might be electronically linked only to other scientists in her area of expertise. She might travel frequently to other places
and countries, covering many miles, and still rarely leave the company
of that same set of peers. Materials and funds might flow into her part
of the suburbs from distant places, but the organizations providing that
material support might be protected from the forces of change by their
size and the depth and age of their bureaucratic structures and from
the demands of the marketplace by massive government or university
funding. Far from inhabiting a section of the city linked to transformations going on elsewhere, such a scientist might be greatly insulated
and so in effect be occupying a rigid and unchanging portion of the
landscape.

    In contrast, residents of the metaphoric "old city" might actually be
inhabiting an exposed cusp of the landscape, where they would feel
acutely the raw impact of forces of change. Although they might not
communicate with fellow professionals in Japan, they might spend
some hours each day contending with images and information from

and about extremely diverse parts of the world. Although they might live in the old city, with its "ancient tangle of received practices, accepted beliefs, habitual judgements, and untaught emotions" (Geertz 1983a:74), they might work each day with others who, probably in diverse ways, have been directly and materially affected by processes of change that are international in origin. They might have lost a job in a steel plant as the economic base of the region shifts from industrial production to service and finance. They might have experienced several rounds of retraining either offered on the job or forced by the loss of a job. They might have moved in and out of the paid workforce several times and from place to place within it, trying to keep body and soul together as the world seems to shift and reconfigure itself. These are not experiences of conservatism and stability. They are experiences of rapid and constant change.

This schematic sketch of hypothetical possibilities is not meant to summarize what my material reveals. As we will see, the actual landscape is more complicated still. Rather, this sketch is meant only to begin to dislodge a common presupposition — that scientists occupy positions in the forefront of changes occurring in the society (and in fact are often seen to be responsible for initiating those changes). In fact, research scientists ensconced in universities, including anthropologists, may be the last to learn about some of the profound shifts shaking most of our major institutions.

Within this topographical image of culture as an old city with modern suburbs, we can think of the research that lies behind this book as three years of concerted traipsing about this metropolis. Instead of the metaphoric metropolis I explored a real one, the old East Coast city of Baltimore. Instead of wandering around alone, I was accompanied by a stalwart group of graduate students.

To ensure that we crisscrossed the cultural terrain in a variety of different ways, we conducted open-ended interviews on the general topic of health (see Appendix 3) with a significant number of people (over two hundred) who lived in diverse socioeconomic settings and who were neither sick (necessarily) nor scientific experts (necessarily). We picked several appropriate neighborhoods (described in Appendix 1), and the students set about entering into the social life of these neighborhoods by living in them, joining neighborhood associations, attending community meetings, block parties, and festivals, and volunteering to work on neighborhood projects. As they met people through these activities, they arranged interviews as people were willing. Most interviews took place in the person's home (a schematic description of the people interviewed is provided in Appendix 2), and almost all were tape-recorded (always with permission), then transcribed and comprehensively indexed using qualitative data management software. Nearly all the interviews lasted over an hour; many lasted over two hours.

For some purposes, especially in Part III, I have treated the interviews as a collectively produced text, a kind of encyclopedia of what a diverse population thinks is sayable, imaginable, or thinkable about health, illness, the body, and the society. Although the interviews were the product of conversations with me and/or one or another of the graduate students, everyone interviewed was given the chance to reflect at length on the same series of cultural puzzles. What was said can, I think, legitimately be taken as a broad indication of what is considered relevant to these matters in this culture. The interviews also show vividly how general cultural relevance is refracted through the particular circumstances of localized communities occupying a certain position in the larger political-economic order.

In addition, the interviews served as a probe into the culture, in the sense that the open-ended nature of the conversations allowed issues and ways of thinking that we could not anticipate to emerge and be heard. In every case, since the "interviews" were usually part of an ongoing relationship between interviewer and interviewee, the conversations were less like a litmus test, in which the interviewer checked scientifically for the presence of some variable, than like a joint exploration, in which both explored issues of mutual concern and interest interpretively. The people we interviewed were not chosen randomly, in the statistical sense. But the range of communities and settings in which we worked ensured that they would make up a broad cross section of the society. I have tried to be sure that this diversity affects the shape of the analysis by quoting almost all the people interviewed somewhere in the book.

A combination of participation and interviewing allowed us to see, from different angles, aspects of how health or illness is being constituted in several other special realms:

- an allergy clinic;
- a support group for survivors of polio, many of whom now experience the effects of postpolio syndrome;

- a clinical study of HIV seroconversion — the ALIVE (AIDS Link to Intravenous Experiences) study — that has been running since 1988, through which we could talk to people whose main "risk factor" for HIV infection was injectable drug use;
- a class of college students who were taking a course in immunology;
- training courses for workers and managers in corporations teaching new ways of organizing the workforce and new ways of interacting; national, regional, and local conferences training the trainers in these techniques;
- activities of the Rouse Corporation in maintaining the profitability of their development at Baltimore's Inner Harbor and in building and maintaining low-cost housing for Baltimore neighborhoods;
- alternative health clinics and their practitioners.

By becoming involved in all these settings, we sought to put ourselves in places where we would be touched and, we hoped, propelled by the same processes affecting other people in the society. We wanted our fieldwork to fetch us up in what have been called *implosions*, places where different elements of the system come into energetic contact and collapse in on themselves (Baudrillard 1985).

Although I am writing this book on my own, a matter that was agreed among the graduate students and myself early in the project, the ongoing research evolved out of our close collaboration. We met weekly to keep each other posted about significant developments, raise questions about what to pursue and what to drop, or ask for help coping with the daily emotional roller coaster of fieldwork: rejection, anger, fear, affection, fulfillment, or loss. We also undertook to write several papers in collaboration, which will be published separately (see Claeson et al. 1991; Martin et al., in press). Because the corpus of interviews was produced as a collective enterprise, and because the text is already filled with so many names, I have not attributed particular interviews to particular interviewers. Nonetheless, since most of us concentrated our efforts in certain areas, readers can get a general idea who conducted which interviews. Bjorn Claeson did many of the interviews in Stockton, Montclair, Hamilton, Riverdale, and Warren; Wendy Richardson did many of the interviews in Franklin; and Monica Schoch-Spana did many of the interviews in Montgomery. Karen-Sue

Taussig concentrated her efforts on ALIVE participants, corporate employees, and trainers, Laury Oaks on AIDS/HIV activists, and Ariane van der Straten on research scientists and graduate students. I was peripatetic.

There are three special problems of methodology related to this project that I want to discuss before leaving the subject. They are the problem of expertise, the problem of sexual identity, and the problem of being ill.

The problem of expertise took two forms. From time to time in the neighborhood interviews, people felt as if they were being tested on subjects about which they had limited knowledge. In spite of the students' and my eloquent (and accurate) statements that we were not experts in biology or medicine either, such is the authority of science and medicine in this society that sometimes these assurances were not enough. One man was worried about sounding like a dummy and wanted Monica to correct him. Another, when asked what he thought of the interview, said he liked how open ended it was but wanted us to contact him later to correct anything he might have got wrong. But these problems were few and far between; almost all the time, the students' appreciative response to whatever people said seemed sufficient to prompt a flood of confident talk. Many people said that they liked the open-ended nature of the questions, that it made them feel important. One man gave us a high compliment, although he surely did not intend it as such. He said, "You're a goddamn alien! These are weird questions!!" The interview made the experts stretch, too. Many scientists we interviewed commented that the questions brought out aspects of their work that they do not usually think about, and, with mixed feelings, we heard one scientist tell us, "Whoever came up with the questions knew enough to ask the right ones."

The problem of sexual identity affected each of us differently. AIDS is an epidemic that devastated the gay community in this country first, and the gay and lesbian community was extraordinarily active and successful in mobilizing education to prevent transmission. In addition, this community was able to influence the questions that scientific researchers were asking and to garner social and material support for HIV+ people. Hence, for all these reasons, there is a special link between the gay and lesbian community and the epidemic.

Each of us working on this project had a different relationship to this community via his or her individual sexual (and other) identities and past experiences. We could no more eliminate these differences or "control" for them than we could cease to be people. What we could and did try to do was to be aware of how our own feelings and attitudes might be affecting our experiences and the reactions of others to us.

The research sometimes led us into the presence of people who were sick and possibly dying: similarly, each of us brought a personal, complicated history of experience with sickness and death to those situations. Among anthropologists, the question of whether those who are HIV– can speak adequately on behalf of those who are HIV+ is a difficult one.[2] I would want to honor the special insights that can come from anthropologists who share a crucial experience of this kind with people in the fieldwork setting. But our fieldwork setting included people with many other life-threatening conditions and many who regarded themselves as basically healthy. This book is not intended principally to communicate the experience of being HIV+, of having AIDS, or being ill; it is intended to explore how, as all of us begin to think of having this thing called *an immune system*, the logic of health, of sickness, and of fitness for survival is changing.[3] Throughout, my effort has been to describe not primarily *what* the experience of being HIV+ or of having an otherwise compromised immune system is like, but *how* it came to be that we now see illness and health in terms of the immune system in the first place.[4]

Since my research has revealed that dramatic shifts in fundamental concepts are under way, it follows that a major amount of effort in the book will go toward providing a historical context in which these shifts can be understood. What were earlier commonsense ideas about health, bodies, and disease that can help us understand the direction that these changes are taking? To provide an answer, I look in detail in Part II at everyday concepts and practices concerning health and the body that prevailed in the 1940s and 1950s.

In addition, in this book I am looking less for a "base of resistance" to domination, a base grounded in something like community, class, gender, or age, than I am for the delicate outlines of an emerging new common sense, entailing changes in notions of identity, groups, wholes, or parts, changes that will have profound implications for how we see all those grounded bases. In fact, many experiences that are characteristic of the current age fly in the face of the spatial image of culture as an old city surrounded by new suburbs that I used at the beginning of this chapter. Among these experiences that seem to defy linear time and space are the "nonplace" of the virtual office (Patton 1993:C1) or the cyberspace of the Internet, "everywhere and nowhere" (Benedikt 1991:1). As evidence of how widespread access to the Internet is becoming, the Maryland state-organized computer link to the Internet, "Seymour," was recording nearly four thousand log-ons per month, even *before* its phone numbers had been made public or it was considered online (Langfitt 1993:4A).

Nor will I be beginning with the expected terms of anthropological analysis: *culture, metaphor, meaning, ritual*. One reason for this is that these terms, sometimes distant cousins of their academic anthropological relatives, are already operating actively in the social contexts that I am studying. For a variety of reasons, people are already using them to explain, analyze, and even change the worlds in which they live. Thus, some analytic terms have become themselves in need of analysis.

In focusing on knowledge of the body from a variety of points of view, including the science of immunology, my account relates to other efforts to track the development of rapidly changing conceptions and practices regarding "life." What have been called the *key* sciences for these developments — genetics and immunology — are both potent sites for the study of transformations in fundamental cultural concepts of *life, person, society*. Paul Rabinow argues that the new genetics will be "an infinitely greater force for reshaping society and life than was the revolution in physics, because it will be embedded throughout the social fabric at the microlevel by medical practices" (1992a:241).[5] In what follows, we will see the beginning of this reshaping in relation to immunology.

I begin in the book as I began in the research, by looking at how people in a variety of social settings talk about health, illness, and the makeup of their bodies. In Part III, I look for the kinds of things that people are able to say about these topics, the underlying grammar of what people bring to such a discussion. The emphasis here is on delineating both the commonalities and the differences among people who have various kinds of experience and expertise. The emphasis is also on seeing how the emerging set of ideas about these topics compares with the common sense of the decades before 1970.

In Part IV, I turn to clusters of ideas and practices, which I will call *configurations*. Each of them leads out into the settings and institutions of the wider society — the state, political organizations, multinational corporations. I have called these clusters *configurations* to try to capture the sense in which they involve ways of thinking and ways of acting simultaneously. They are ways of seeing the world attached to forms of patterned activity that are social in character.[6] The term points to a pattern or shape (more or less fuzzy) that is simultaneously how we see the world and a result of how the social world is ordered.

Finally, in Part V, I shift my focus from configurations to processes through which these configurations are generated. I have called these processes *practicums* for two reasons. First, I want to evoke, but distinguish these processes from, what the sociologist Pierre Bourdieu called the *habitus*. For Bourdieu, the *habitus* refers to dispositions laid down in early childhood, patterns that make it possible for people to live in a world filled with taken-for-granted meanings, that ordinarily need neither close analysis, conscious purposefulness, nor adherence to a set of rules (Bourdieu 1977:80–81).

My focus will be on *change* rather than on *habit*, on processes from which people learn that may *not* have been in place since childhood and processes that may contain a degree of intention on the part of those wishing to perpetuate them. "Practicums" involve learning about new concepts of the ideal and fit person, often in noninstitutional settings. I mean to imply learning, but learning that is often less formally structured than it would be in a school. As often as not, the practicums that I discuss seem to us already to be an ordinary, mundane part of daily life, not a special exercise in a special class that we attend. Even where practicums are used inside an institution, such as a corporation, the complex combination of physical and psychological experiences evoked often means that the "teachers" are not exactly in control of the outcome. I also mean to imply learning that is embedded in some sort of complex physical-mental experience.

A second reason for the choice of the term *practicum* will become clear only as the book unfolds: a variety of domains (concepts of health, the body, survival) conspire together to bring to the foreground particular contemporary notions of *training* and *education*, notions that draw on the specifically American connection between education and liberal democracy. These notions are as powerful for what they evoke about the equal potential of all humans to learn as for what they conceal. As we will see, what they conceal is that, for lack of resources, not everyone can obtain the same quality or amount of training or education; what they also conceal is that, even given ample education and training, the task that must be learned (the ability to adapt to constant change) is such that some will inevitably fail or refuse to learn.

Speaking of the development of ideas and practices attached to microbes and the hygiene needed to control them in the nineteenth century, Bruno Latour remarks that he is less interested in the *"application"* of a given power such as hygiene "on the bodies of the wretched and the poor" than in "the earlier *composition* of an unpredictable source of power. It is precisely at the time when no one can tell whether he is dealing with a new source of power that the link between science and society is most important. When almost everyone is convinced, then, but only then and afterward, will hygiene be a 'power' to discipline and to coerce" (1988:256). This book describes the era *after* the era of hygiene, at a time when immune systems thinking is "nudging" hygiene over to make room for itself. Many people are in the process of becoming convinced, but by no means everyone is already convinced. The complex of immune system concepts and practices that I will describe is *emergent*.

Broad as the agenda for this book is, I am very aware that there are central parts of my research with which I have dealt only tangentially. One of these, restructuring in the organization of work, I treat briefly in Chapter 11; another, processes that involve the development of new norms of health and new kinds of normalization, I touch on in the conclusion. Both form the core of a second volume that I am in the process of writing.

Readers who know my earlier work about reproductive biology may be wondering whether I will cast the science of immunology in the role of the villainous creator of a new imagery of domination. In the research for this book, I have found that it is hard to name the villain when I have observed a set of organizing ideas with similar potential implications operating in departments of immunology and departments of anthropology — or when the head of the human resource department in my own university uses exactly the same language, and is planning the same sort of group activities, as many managers of industrial corporations in the region and as indeed those of us who teach may well have used in the classroom to liberate learning from its old hierarchical constraints.

Even though the task of finding culprits seems both fruitless and misguided, the implications of the ideas that I discuss in this book do include an emerging sense of an organization of the world that will benefit only certain people. So, even though no one individual, and no one group, is at fault, it is no less important to identify what the emerging "common sense" is and how we come to think of it as natural and desirable.

Japanese society is often held up to Americans as the model to follow if we want to survive successfully in the next century. While such comparisons often suffer from an overly simplified understanding of Japan and as well as of the United States, I think that it is still instructive to see some aspects of Japanese society in relation to some of the principles of action and interaction that are only now emerging in the United States. In her study of political resistance in Japan, "the world's most orderly and prosperous society," Norma Field remarks on how the potency of the Japanese belief in the importance of social harmony leads to denial of conflict in the past and present and to the "repressiveness of everyday life":

> Where there are neither visible oppressors nor victims, and where the memory of historical suffering has grown remote, freedom becomes subtle, banal, and finally, elusive. To call attention to its flight amidst pervasive prosperity is a thankless undertaking. Most who embark on such a venture have not chosen it. They have been driven to it, by vivid confrontation with the residues of historic oppression, by encounters with victims and oppressors, who are, after all, produced even in times of prosperity and peace as well as war, and finally, by recognition of the repressiveness of everyday life, a recognition they cannot dispel in spite of the potency of common sense, most especially the belief in the existence and importance of social harmony. (Field 1991:28)

In quoting Field out of context, I run the risk of reducing her nuanced account to a simple caricature of Japan as a totalitarian society that represses freedom. Her book conveys a far more subtle picture of Japan than this: it is her complex description of how ideals of harmony are simultaneously accepted and questioned by the Japanese that most illuminates what is going on in the United States.

As we will see vividly in the following pages, the "pervasive prosperity" that Field finds in Japan does not characterize the United States following the Reagan-Bush years: suffering from hunger, disease, and homelessness is located in the recent past and present for many people.[7] In the face of this, we are frequently told that certain changes are necessary if the United States is to achieve a new, inclusive prosperity — such changes as restructuring corporations to make them smaller, leaner, and more agile or restructuring the workforce to make it more flexible and able to adapt to constant change. Yet adopting the very measures that seem so compellingly necessary to achieve a new, inclusive prosperity may entail a dampening of social conflict as we learn to adjust and adapt for the sake of the whole. Here, as in Japan, taking on the values of social harmony to assure prosperity for all could lead to an extraordinary repressiveness of everyday life. It is most fundamentally against this possibility that I have written this book.

One caveat is necessary before I proceed. I began this research in 1989, the first year of the Bush administration. Most of what I describe about impending or ongoing changes in fundamental concepts of bodies and selves I observed during the next three years, all Bush years. During Bush's fourth year in office, the political campaign that led to the election of Bill Clinton suddenly placed an extensive rhetoric of "change" on every campaign television ad, in every television talk show, and every news report. As Clinton gained visibility and credibility and finally won, I experienced an eerie feeling. The people who were advising him, the books he read, and the authorities he cited in his own writings were often the very people who, operating very much in the background of a Republican administration, had been the dominant spokespersons for the changes I was studying in the realm of corporate organization and health care. It was these very people whose visions of the ideal person, organization, and society were resonating so strongly with what I was discovering in other domains, such as science, and in the health conceptions of ordinary people in all walks of life.[8] During the second presidential debate, someone asked Clinton whether he intended to raise taxes on the middle class. I heard him reply, "No, but the middle classes will have their jobs cut out for them anyway: they will have to get used to continuous education and retraining if they are going to be able to compete in the new society that must be forged." All of a sudden, I saw the ethnographic material that I had been gathering as a kind of rising sea that had been surging powerfully around but had had no national focus or spokesperson. Clinton's team of experts, whose influence had been limited to the domains of industry and education, now had a national forum: the rising sea may become a tidal wave. What my research shows is that, whatever form the tidal wave takes, it will be the crest of a sea made up of a public awareness far more extensive than the voices of a few experts.

PART
TWO

HISTORICAL OVERVIEW

Even in the flattest landscape there are passes where the road first climbs to a peak and then descends into a new valley. Most of these passes are only topography, with little or no difference in climate, language, or culture between the valleys on either side. But some passes are different. They are true divides. They often are neither high nor spectacular. The Brenner is the lowest and gentlest of the passes across the Alps; yet from earliest times it has marked the border between Mediterranean and Nordic cultures. . . . History, too, knows such divides. They also tend to be unspectacular and are rarely much noticed at the time. But once these divides have been crossed, the social and political landscape changes. Social and political climate is different and so is social and political language. There are new realities.

PETER DRUCKER, *The New Realities*

As I trace the shape of the body landscape on either side of the divide, we will find that sometimes the two sides coexist in tension with each other, the way a traveler's memory of past experiences can inform his or her experiences of the present. In our technical and everyday concepts and practices concerning health and the body, the old landscape on the far side of the divide lives on, called into salience from time to time by a variety of new circumstances met on the near side.

I am aware that, in drawing such a division between past and present, I risk falling into serious traps: surrounding the past with a nostalgic yearning for a lost utopia or surrounding the present with the redemptive capacity to compensate for what was lacking in the past.[1] In my case, I have some protection from feeling nostalgic about health in the 1940s and 1950s: as I mentioned earlier, my brother died of polio during an epidemic in 1951. When I pore over popular magazine articles about health and illness from that time, my flesh crawls. Photographs of quarantine signs for polio bring to mind the yellow placard on my front door; lists of ways to avoid polio bring to mind all the things I mortally feared as a child. These childhood experiences, however, give me no protection against bestowing redemptive qualities on aspects of the present.

To begin by looking back, what might everyday understandings of the body have been like at the end of the first half of the century in the United States? For my review of this period, I rely on popular

health manuals and home health books primarily from the 1940s and
1950s and popular periodicals such as the *Ladies' Home Journal* and
Time, also from this period. I have also used a remarkable study conducted in 1955 under the auspices of the National Opinion Research
Center (NORC) and based on 2,379 intensive personal interviews, for
which the original forms, with replies recorded in longhand, still survive in the NORC archives in Chicago.[2]

Early twentieth-century ideas about health reflected the impact of
the new science of bacteriology, which brought laboratory techniques
to bear on the attempt to understand the role of microorganisms in
causing disease.[3] Some historians of medicine have argued that the
influence of bacteriology reduced the scope of public health concerns
from the broad, morally informed programs that were common in
nineteenth-century public health activities to narrower, more technical concerns focused on what could be revealed in microscopes and
test tubes (Starr 1982:196).[4] Others have argued that, although bacteriology "narrowed the theoretical underpinnings of contagious disease
control" and elevated the importance of laboratory procedures, in the
early twentieth century it largely did not "contract the comprehen-
siveness of public health work in contagious disease control": "Early
twentieth-century proponents of bacteriology could no more isolate
disease from its environmental and social context than could their pre-
decessors who were driven by the filth theory of disease" (Leavitt
1992:629).[5] But, by the 1940s and 1950s, the focus of public health
thinking had narrowed. Whereas in earlier decades the condition of
the whole city, for example, would have been of concern, by this time
people were more apt to think in terms of the cleanliness of their own
immediate environment, their own house and their bodies.[6]

In the 1940s and 1950s, seen through the lens of popular publications, the most important threats to health were considered to lie in
the environment just outside the body. Enormous attention was devoted to hygiene, cleaning surfaces in the home, clothing, surfaces of
the body and wounds with antiseptics. The cleanliness recommendations of the National Foundation for Infantile Paralysis were widely
publicized: "Good personal health habits help prevent the disease from
spreading. Wash hands before eating, before handling food. Teach
children not to exchange bites of candy, not to put dirty hands or
objects into their mouths. Keep flies and other insects away from food"
("Help Prevent Infantile Paralysis" 1948:89). "Pay attention to all the
minute details of cleanliness" (Bernsley 1951:6). A mother of fourteen

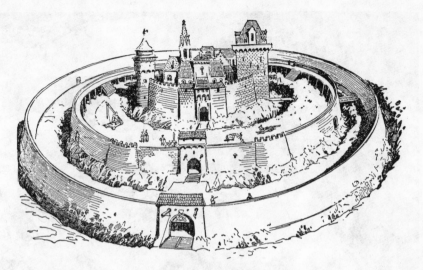

Fig. 1. *The castle of health — an early twentieth-century view of the healthy body protected behind castle walls. From J. W. Ritchie,* Primer of Sanitation and Physiology *(1918:16).*

children recalled how she had followed these rules: "[She] made all of them, over loud protest, wash themselves thoroughly before every meal. 'They were real clean before they ate,' she recalls" (Schriftgiesser 1952:18). Nonetheless, eleven of her children contracted polio.

Even though, in cases like that of this family, hygiene seemed to fail, sanitary measures were frequently linked to the presence of microbes, the object being to keep them from entering the body. If polio is to be prevented, it was advised, "only clean things should enter the mouth when polio is around, since the virus probably enters the body through the mouth" (Gross 1949:131). Advertisements for cleaning compounds stressed the presence of "deadly disease germs *by the millions* [that] may lurk unseen in ordinary house dust": Lysol (and others) were "potent, germ-killing," and could clean *"hygienically"* (*Ladies' Home Journal*, February 1947,156).

The most important defense was strictly preventing the entrance of any germs into the interior of the body (Clark and Cumley 1953:103). This notion was clearly already present in imagery from the early decades of the century. In an illustration of "the castle of health" (see fig. 1), *The Primer of Sanitation and Physiology* shows the lines of defense against disease (Ritchie 1918:16).[7] The two outer defenses are, "Keep germs from being spread about," and, "Guard the gateways by

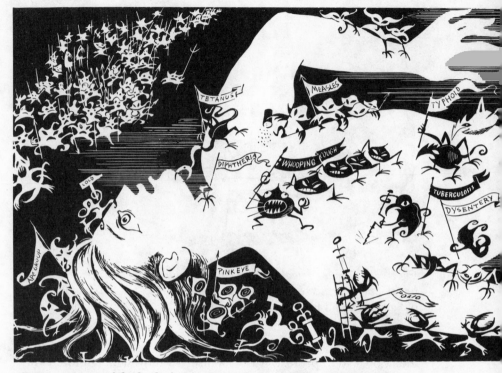

Fig. 2. *A view of the body from 1955 with the "liliputian hordes" of germs and viruses trying to penetrate the seamless surface of the body. From R. Coughlan, "Science Moves in on Viruses,"* Life, *20 June 1955, 122.*

which they enter the body." The castle itself represents the body, into which the illustration does not let us see at all, and which is dwarfed by the much larger outer defenses.

By the 1940s and 1950s, the body seems to have become even more elaborately defended at its surface. An illustration from a 1955 article on polio in *Life* (see fig. 2) shows the body as a seamless whole, its surface besieged by germs of all sorts, some drilling away with drill bits, and some slain and marked by the victory flags of effective vaccines (Coughlan 1955:122–23). An ad for Listerine in 1947 attests to its ability to kill germs on the *surface* of the mouth and throat and asserts, "The time to strike a cold is at its very outset . . . to go after the surface germs before they go after you" (*Ladies' Home Journal*, January 1947, 9). An elementary school textbook warns, "*Be on Guard at All Times.* You must be on guard at all times. Disease germs are always on hand to

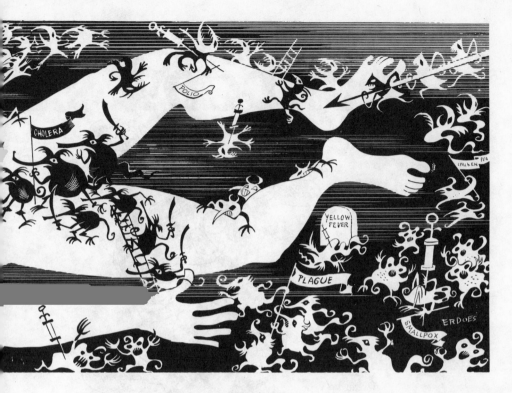

attack. Be clean in everything you do. Remember, you must keep your hair and scalp, your fingernails and toenails, and your clothing clean as well as your skin. Keep fighting to destroy disease germs. Form habits that will protect you from harm" (Burkard, Chambers, and Maroney 1950:42).

While researching this chapter, I found myself tripped up more than once by my own assumptions from the present that did not adequately take into account the significance of body surfaces and openings in the 1940s and 1950s. For example, many articles on preventing polio mention that one should avoid having tonsils or teeth removed during the summer polio season. I unthinkingly assumed that this was to avoid additional stress that could generally weaken the body's defenses. I was brought up short when an article in the *Woman's Home Companion* spelled out what was probably obvious to people at that time: the removal of tonsils and teeth leaves raw nerve ends that could serve as an entry point for the polio virus (Ratcliff 1947:34–35). It was the opening left in the body's surfaces — a literal physical breach — that would allow disease to get in.

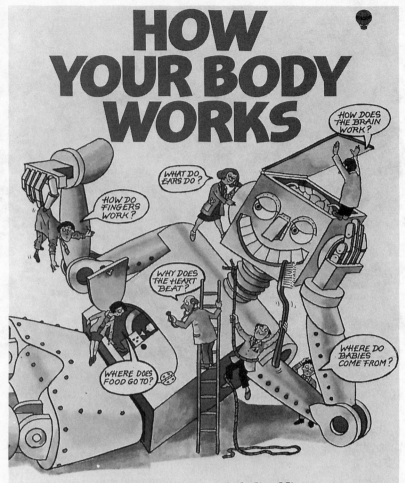

Fig. 3. *The body as machine. From the cover of J. Hindley and C. King,* How Your Body Works *(1975). Reprinted with permission of Usborne Publishing Ltd.*

Images of the body as a machine abound during this period (see fig. 3).[8] For example, "An optimistic view of life . . . acts on the body like oil on the working of machinery . . . it prevents friction" (Peabody and Hunt 1934:374). The body's efficiency is measured and compared to that of industrial machines (Clark and Cumley 1953:69). "The human body is a machine, amenable to the same chemical and physical laws as most of the machines man makes himself for his own ends." The cells of the body are "disciplined," "like the City during working hours"; the organs and limbs of the body are nourished by the body's blood just as the workers in a busy factory depend on the surrounding community for their nourishment (Wells, Huxley, and Wells 1939:24, 44–45).

In accord with the machine model, the body is seen as made up of parts that can break down: in the NORC interviews, people refer to illness in terms of a body part: "ear trouble," "kidney trouble," "stomach trouble," "suffering with my back," "my tonsils," "my kidneys." The body emerges as a machine that sometimes requires overhaul: "We get a complete going over by the company doctor every year even our eyes examined. I'm a street car motorman and they don't take any chances on our health."

Although the parts of the body can be fixed so that it can once again function smoothly, there is, in strong contrast to what we will find later, very little sense of anything that holds the whole body together. There is frequent use of the term *system* as in "gentle to the system" (of a laxative), "his system has thrown off the virus" (of polio), "vaccines help the system build antibodies" (of the Salk vaccine), or "your system ain't always in a good condition for [a drink]" (NORC survey). But in every case the term could be replaced simply by *body* or a personal pronoun. *System* works here, in contrast to later periods, as an all-purpose term that can stand in for any body function.[9]

The "supreme importance" of regular, predictable habits is stressed (Peabody and Hunt 1934:621), the good habits of personal hygiene as well as the good habits learned by cells to produce antibodies (Clendening 1930:351). "The habits of healthy living taught in the modern school — varied and adequate diet, sufficient sleep, exercise, recreation and mental hygiene — should play a vital part in the development of a healthy mind and body" ("Have You a Health Conscience?" 1952:70). Schoolchildren are guided by a poem:

> *GOOD HABITS — GOOD HEALTH*
> *To win the game of health, you'll need*
> *Good habits by the score.*
> *They are true friends to you indeed,*
> *So each day add one more.*
> (Burkard, Chambers, and Maroney 1950:17)

The notion of automatic habits as one's "true friends" fits comfortably with the notion of the external agents of disease, viruses or bacteria, as active agents, to which the body passively responds. "Immunity" is "induced" in the body. Immunity "is believed to reside chiefly in the circulating blood and its production *is stimulated by* certain unknown, probably protein, constituents of the virus" (Howe 1951a:41; emphasis added). Similarly, vaccines work by stimulating the body to produce antibodies (Engel 1955).

Not only schools advocated hygienic habits. Henry Ford, architect of the work process most characteristic of the time, the moving assembly line organized for mass production, sent investigators into workers' homes to scrutinize their private lives. Over one hundred investigators visited workers' homes and admonished them to practice thrifty and hygienic habits and avoid smoking, gambling, and drinking. These early social workers decided which workers "because of unsatisfactory personal habits or home conditions" were not eligible to receive the full five-dollar wage that Ford offered (Gelderman 1981:56–57).[10] Specifically targeting worker families of foreign birth, the company deplored foreigners' predilection for " 'dark, ill-ventilated and foul-smelling' rooms, and their disregard of the cardinal virtue of cleanliness practiced by 'the most advanced people' " (Banta 1993:213).

When the general notion of *resistance* comes up, it is a kind of passive resistance, the way a solid wall can "resist" being knocked down. Often the emphasis is on the way a person just is, rather than on what he or she has done to build up resistance: "Those fortunate people who never get emotionally upset or physically overfatigued seldom catch cold, no matter how frequently they are exposed" (Lobsenz 1954:54). To further dampen any thought that one could actively increase one's resistance, evidence that was widely circulated in the press in the 1950s led to the conclusion that building up the individual's natural resistance through diet and hygiene was not effective in fighting virus diseases. Scientists found that, in animals, malnutrition led to increased resistance (Howe 1951b:37). Just how far the common sense of that time was from today's is revealed in the astonished reaction to a glimpse of the future: in 1954 *Time* reported on a "radically new approach" to disease, described in a "vision of the future" by René Dubos: "The power to resist infectious disease will be built into, and maintained in, man himself" ("Vision of the Future" 1954:78).

This body whose surfaces are its best protection against disease does not have much going for it inside. Almost none of the periodical articles on health or illness depict processes inside the body graphically. Occasionally reference is made to "fighting" disease, but the elaborated images of military defenses inside the body that we will see emerging later in time are simply not there. When military terms are used in reference to disease at this time, they refer to medical teams, public health organizations, or the National Foundation for Infantile Paralysis (O'Connor 1949).

Only in 1954, after gamma globulin became widely available shortly before the Salk vaccine was produced, did popular periodicals turn their attention to what might be going on inside the body. Gamma globulin is that fraction of human blood that consists of antibodies; gamma globulin from the blood of many donors is combined to increase the likelihood that any dose will contain antibodies against polio. The hope is that these borrowed antibodies will confer a temporary immunity. That year, there was widespread coverage of what "antibodies" are. Here is *Parents' Magazine*'s version: "Antibodies are one of nature's most important ways of protecting animals and men from infectious diseases. When your body is invaded by disease germs . . . it responds by producing antibodies which have a sort of lock-and-key relationship to the invading particles. Though powerless against other germs, these antibodies have a unique ability to 'latch onto' the germs they fit and render them harmless" (Brecher and Brecher 1954:31). Talk of antibodies and how they work in relation to other entities within the body provides a glimpse around a corner into future interpretations of the body in which, as we will see, antibodies will be only one of many denizens of the body charged with warding off disease.

The late 1940s and 1950s were times of heightened middle-class domesticity, as women were forced out of jobs they had held during the war and families often settled in newly burgeoning but isolated and commodity-oriented suburbs.[11] A house, children, a husband, and all their clothes and other things needed to be kept hygienically clean; commodities of cleanliness, from Lysol to an automatic washer, became the housewife's companions. In "Levittowns" built after the war, Bendix washing machines were included in the purchase price (Jackson 1985).

From inside the safe and clean home, the world outside looked dangerous and hostile. Hunkered down in low-slung houses surrounded by fences, housewives were exhorted by the government to prepare for nuclear emergency, learn skills that would be useful in case of an atomic attack, and stock a home bomb shelter (May 1988:103–8). And, of course, home health books of the sort described above often contained sections on this hazard to health. *The Family Physician* (Pomeranz and Koll 1957) has "Protecting Yourself against an Atomic Bomb" as its last chapter, complete with a pictorial section on precautions and first aid (see fig. 4).[12] Fear and anxieties about instantaneous "collective annihilation" from external enemies armed with atom bombs (Boyer 1985:278) and internal traitors who might aid and abet them (Boyer 1985:278; Heale 1990) permeated the age.

After the 1940s and 1950s, attention to the defenses *within* the body increases exponentially. In books written in the 1960s and 1970s, we begin to find accounts of safeguards within the body that come into operation if the "outer fortifications" (the skin or mucous membranes) are breeched. If that should happen, inside the body a whole "new series of defenses goes into action" (Miller and Goode 1960:54–55). In one illustrated book for children, the body is again shown as a castle, complete with a moat, turrets, and armed soldiers to protect it from

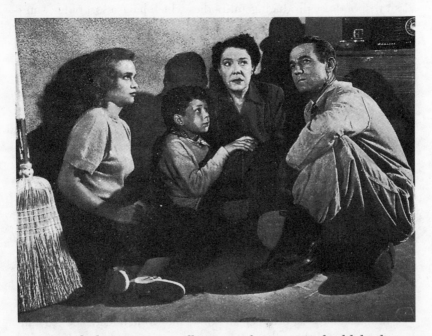

Fig. 4. *In the basement — an illustration from a 1950s health book showing a family taking shelter from an atomic attack. From H. Pomeranz and I. S. Koll,* The Family Physician *(1957:following p. 526).*

germs (see fig. 5). But the shift from the earlier illustration in *Life* is made plain in the cutaway view of what is inside the castle walls. Through the breach in the wall, we can see rank upon rank of soldiers stretching back *inside* the body, ready to fight any germs that might enter (Hindley and King 1975:34–35).

As the interior comes into focus, concern with hygiene and the cleanliness of the outside surfaces of the body diminishes. It is as if, whatever is out there, and however deadly and dirty it is, the body's interior lines of defense will be able to handle it.[13] By the time we reach accounts in contemporary biology and health books, as we will see in detail later, the interior of the body has been enormously elaborated. "Recognition" of disease-causing microbes is fantastically honed and refined, and the immune system "tailors" highly specific responses that can be almost unimaginably various. Drawing on an immense, genetically generated, and constantly changing arsenal of resources, the body can hardly rely on mere habit any longer.

IN THIS SKETCH of changing sensibilities about the body, I have relied so far on the tracings of these changes in popular literature and in the voices of those citizens interviewed by NORC. Is there a similar transition in the perceptions of scientists? Fortunately for me, immunologists of the past have numerous chroniclers. Take, for example, the recent definitive history of the discipline, *A History of Immunology*, (1989) by Arthur Silverstein, himself an immunologist. According to Silverstein, the story of immunology is the story of several transitions. The first one is the transition from "passive" to "active" theories. In passive theories, the pathogen is seen as acting by itself to produce immunity in an otherwise inert host (p. 18). Until around the turn of the century, almost all theories were passive theories. Then, with the discovery of antibodies in the 1890s, there was a transition to theories involving an active host response.

The second transition is from instruction theories of how antibodies are formed to selection theories. *Instruction* theories, which came into vogue after the large number of antibodies in the blood was recognized, held that the body *learned* how to manufacture new forms of antibodies from new kinds of foreign material (antigens) with which it came into contact, as if "the antigen was incorporated in the cell as a die which stamped its pattern on" the antibody (Burnet 1962:89). After the Second World War, *selection* theories came into prominence to

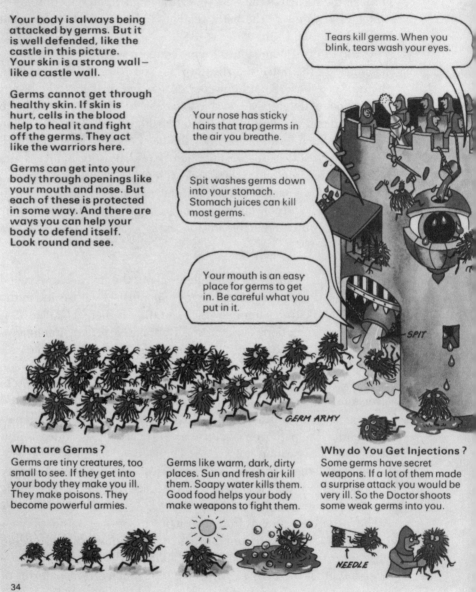

Fig. 5. *The body as a castle, showing, in a cutaway view, the internal ranks of soldiers at the ready inside the body's walls. From J. Hindley*

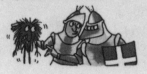

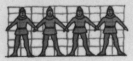

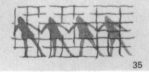

What is a Scab?

Your blood cells learn about the new weapons from the weak germs, and work out how to destroy them. Then you are prepared for an attack.

Part of your blood makes a net when you are cut. Your blood cells bunch up behind it. This makes a blood clot. Dried clotted blood becomes a scab.

The scab protects you while new skin is built. When the new skin is ready, the scab falls off.

and C. King, How Your Body Works *(1975:34–35). Reprinted with permission of Usborne Publishing Ltd.*

account for the large number of antibodies known to be present that could not be accounted for by any known exposure to existing antigens (Silverstein 1989:77). As the immunologist Frank Macfarlane Burnet explained the insights that led to this shift, "[Danish immunologist Neils] Jerne in essence said, 'How do we know that the antigen instructs the cells to produce such and such an antibody? Could it not be that they produce spontaneously a wide variety of potential antibodies and that when an antigen enters the body it is met by one of these natural antibody molecules carrying an appropriate pattern? As a result of this meeting a call goes out for the production of more of this particular sort of antibody'" (Burnet 1962:89–90). One of my immunology lecturers was fond of stressing the immense variety of antibodies by saying that we even have antibodies specific to antigens that would be found only on Mars!

The mechanism posited to account for the presence of all these antibodies was genetic mutation and selection. Through mutation that takes place during the course of life, sometimes called *somatic mutation*, the immune system can produce an astonishing variety of antibodies. (Another lecturer told us that the number of specific types of antibodies that exist at any one time in a human being is now thought to be ten trillion, and the estimate has been going up every year.) This huge repertoire, prepared in advance against any possible eventuality, allows the immune system to be seen as an *anticipatory* system.

The third transition that Silverstein describes involves the increasing importance of the concept of immunological specificity, which came to the fore after 1970 and which forms the central two chapters in Silverstein's book. The nature of the flexible specificity of the immune system can be easily illustrated by an experimental technique: you can oblate the immune system of a mouse by radiation and then inject human bone marrow cells into it. (Bone marrow cells are the precursors of all immune system cells.) In the mouse's body, the human cells will develop into a competent and entirely functional immune system (Bishop 1988). Out of the enormous variety of antibodies being continuously produced by some cells in the immune system, largely B cells, certain antibodies are selected for production in increased quantities. The enormous variety even includes antibodies that only a mouse would need, and transplantation of the human system into a mouse's body triggers the production of more of those antibodies. In sum, the immune system "*first* generates a diverse population of antibody molecules and then selects *ex post facto* those that fit or match. It does this

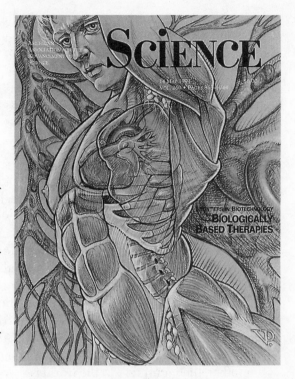

Fig. 6. *A 1993 cover of*
Science *magazine shows*
a body with no skin at all,
the gleaming white
lymph nodes, key parts of
the immune system,
exposed to view.
From Science, *vol. 260,*
14 May 1993. Reprinted
with permission of
Science, © *AAAS.*

continually and, for the most part, adaptively" (Edelman 1992:78).

What we see emerging through the immunologists' eyes by the late twentieth century, then, is a body that actively relates to the world, that actively selects from a cornucopia of continually produced new antibodies that keep the body healthy and enable it to meet every new challenge. Possessed of agile responses, and flexible specificity, our adroit, innovative bodies are poised to anticipate any conceivable challenge.

All these transitions take place within the context of the assumption, which gradually grew more clearly articulated over the 1960s and 1970s, that the various parts of the immune response form a single, interconnected *system* (Moulin 1991:346). This framework resides entirely within the body, where it links the body to its changing environment. In arresting contrast to the 1950s body, the interior hidden behind its protective layer of skin, the 1990s body, as depicted on the cover of *Science*, has no skin at all on its torso (see fig. 6). The protective skin has been stripped away to reveal gleaming white lymph nodes (under the arms and in the groin), key places where immune system cells are trained and mobilized. This is a literally muscled being, with the face of a Greek god and the pose of a dancer, a depiction whose significance will come to light in due course.

Before moving to a detailed consideration of comparable shifts in popular conceptions of the body after the 1970s in the next chapter, I want to point out that the people we interviewed also saw the broad outlines of such a shift in thinking about the body. A biology professor graphically describes the shift as he sees it:[14]

> In terms of personal empowerment, the idea that we have this thing [the immune system], we don't even know it's working, we don't have to know it's working, it's always taking care of us, it's always doing these amazing things to keep us well. I think it's very empowering to think about the immune system, like we are strong. We are powerful. We are protected. We have almost like the scientific version of thinking about an angel or a protector or something that they probably did in the Middle Ages. And it's us, and we're really strong. I think people who don't think about the immune system walk around saying, Oh God, this farm is all full of germs. My mother, for example, my mother and my grand-mother, their attitude was the world is very dangerous and there are all these germs and what if we get them. I mean they never ever thought in terms of, well, we're strong, we get them every day. And we beat them. (Peter Keller)

A midwife perceives the difference between thinking of health as maintained by internal processes and thinking of it as related to uncon-nected factors from the outside.

> *What's your conception of how the immune system works?*
> *Or what the immune system is?*
> It is our defense against disease.
> *Is that how you think of it?*
> I see it as sort of what keeps us in balance, or kind of keeps us well, but I think it is that thing that sort of helps us to fight off foreign whatevers, when they come into our system, you know, it's what keeps the colds away, it's what keeps the cancer cells from becoming a big problem, it's what keeps us healthy, basi-

cally. A monitoring system, and a defense system at the same
time.

*Do you think that your parents thought about a system like
that?*

[Laughs.] No. Do I think they even knew what an immune system was? No.

*Or even thought about some kind of a defense system like
that?*

I don't think so. I mean they really were of the era of vaccines,
you know, the polio vaccine, everybody ran out and got their
sugar cubes, and of the four basic food groups. I mean that's
sort of where they came from with health, take a vitamin every
day, eat four basic food groups, get your immunization, and
you're set to go, and I don't know if they ever really put it all
together. . . . I don't know really if they ever sat down and
thought about how that all worked in their systems. (Katherine
Johnson)

An employee of an AIDS service organization and an employee of a
local dairy discuss how the importance of hygiene has waned since
their parents' time:

*Do you think your parents' generation thought about the
immune system?*

CK: I think yes. I don't think they called it that. It was like they
have good blood, or they come from good stock, but the
immune system per se, they didn't label that.

LR: I don't think they thought about the immune system.

CK: Well, you came from a family of long livers, or short
livers.

LR: They must have thought of germs, because you know, in the
fifties and sixties especially, disinfectants and cleansers were
big. Very, very big. And when you think of all the laundry and
all the cleaning our mothers did. . . . But I think they connected
it with germs. I think the focus was on germs. I don't think that
they focused on the immune system at all. I think it was germs
and medicine. I think that the immune system was really left
out. I don't remember my mother mentioning the immune system, or an adult mentioning the immune system. It was germs

had to be killed before they could even get to you. That's how
bad germs were.
CK: Yeah, that's when they came out with the vaccines and
everything. So if the germ accidentally got into your body, you
would have the vaccine to kill it before it did any harm. (Cindy
Kessler and Lynn Ritchie)

The magnitude of the contemporary shift in body imagery that we
have begun to glimpse in the statements reported above might lead us
to wonder whether it is happening in connection with some major shift
in the social order. Certainly, many political economists are trying to
describe a major shift in the forces of production that began in the
1970s. This shift, associated with late capitalism and often termed *flexible specialization*, has been called "the signature of a new economic
epoch" (Borgmann 1992:75).[15] The "flexibility" in this new shape of the
economy refers both to labor and to products: labor markets become
more variable over time as workers move in and out of the workforce
more rapidly; the process of labor itself varies too, workers taking on
managerial tasks and managers spending time on the assembly floor,
as dictated by changing production conditions. Products also become
more flexible: design processes grow more versatile and technology
more able rapidly to adapt to the needs of production. *Specialization*
refers to the custom marketing of goods produced cheaply in small
batches for particular customers ("tailor-made" production) and the
consequent decline of mass production and standardized products
(Smith 1991:139).
    The acceleration in the pace of product innovation, together with
the exploration of highly specialized and small-scale market niches,
spawns new organizational forms such as the "just-in-time" inventory-
flows delivery system, which cuts down radically on stocks required to
keep production flow going (Harvey 1989:156). Laborers experience a
speedup in the processes of labor and an intensification in the retraining that is constantly required. New technologies in production reduce
turnover time dramatically, entailing similar accelerations in exchange
and consumption. "Improved systems of communication and information flow, coupled with rationalizations in techniques of distribution
(packaging, inventory control, containerization, market feed-back, etc.)
make it possible to circulate commodities through the market system
with greater speed" (p. 285). Time and space are compressed, as the
time horizons of decision making shrink and instantaneous communi-

cation and cheaper transport costs allow decisions to be effected over a global space (p. 147). Multinational capital operates in a globally integrated environment: ideally, capital flows unimpeded across all borders, all points are connected by instantaneous communication, and products are made as needed for the momentary and continuously changing market.[16]

The people we interviewed, who speak often in the following pages, have become involved in these processes in complex ways, as, like other old East Coast cities, Baltimore experiences the wrenching consequences of the increasing concentration of capital, both nationally and globally, and the decline of its former manufacturing sector: "population drain, increased poverty, an income gap between city and suburban residents, gaps among racial groups, long-term unemployment . . . , homelessness, hunger, low education levels, high crime rates, and very high taxes" (Zukin 1991a:245; see also Meyers 1986).

Baltimore is classified as a regional center for "diversified services," which include providing headquarters, services for producers, distributive services, as well as nonprofit and government activities. Consequently, while it is experiencing very heavy losses of manufacturing jobs, the city is also experiencing "at least matching gains within key services" (Noyelle and Stanback 1984:53).[17] Still, the overall direction during the years of this study was toward increasing unemployment and poverty.[18]

Seeking to rebuild a viable social space, cities like Baltimore have, among other things, attempted to attract capital investment in renewed downtown centers. Using the attractions of restored nineteenth-century architecture and a waterfront, Baltimore, like Boston and many other cities, constructed a spectacular attraction called the Inner Harbor.[19] It is a "permanent commercial 'festival' " designed to attract middle-class residents and tourists back to the center of the city (Zukin 1991b:257). In the process, inevitably, housing, shops, and jobs for the poor of the inner city have been displaced (p. 258). New jobs produced for local residents, both in the "festival" itself and in the supporting hotels, corporate headquarters, and finance centers, are likely to be low-paying service jobs.[20] In the novel *Red Baker*, Red, who was a skilled steelworker in a Baltimore mill that has shut down, faces the specter of a public works job at the Inner Harbor: "Yeah, I got the picture. . . . My wife is working as a waitress in Weaver's Crab House, and she looks out the window and sees me, her husband, bagging trash, crab claws, and french fries people have thrown out. Picking up candy wrappers and ice cream sticks. You think I'm going to be able to hack that?" (Ward 1985:30).[21]

There was an acute awareness among many people we interviewed that, although the extravagant development in Baltimore's Inner Harbor had pulled in external sources of capital investment through its spectacular attractions, it had dubious long-term economic benefits for city residents. Before the harbor was developed "there were warehouses on the harbor, warehouses that were about to fall down, and there were oil slicks in the water and dead fish floating around, and nobody wanted to go to the inner harbor. . . . But all of a sudden, people are paddle boating out in the water, and they're having balloon ascensions, and everybody's going down there to eat hot dogs and pizza, and it's like, what a change. . . . I think it's great. It's about time, because Baltimore was really going down the tubes. Don't you think?" (Daryl Huff). But, as John Parker put it, the city may be "cosmetically vibrant," but the truth is a lot uglier. Mildred Cosgrove agreed:

[The mayor] was saying the city was in such excellent condition and the city was doing OK, and he still stressed, We're doing this at the Inner Harbor, we're doing that at the Inner Harbor! People don't want to hear that, because the average citizen here in Baltimore, they don't go to the Inner Harbor. It's a tourist attraction. They're not interested in the Harbor, they're interested in getting their neighborhoods straightened out, you know? And as far as I'm concerned, the Inner Harbor, you can take it and sink it. . . . [The mayor wants] to lay off five hundred city employees, and he said the city is doing fine; it's not doing fine. . . . There's no way in the world if I was a city employee you could tell me the city's doing fine when I went to work Monday morning and I got a pink slip. No way.

The attractions of the Inner Harbor could not outweigh experiences of increased unemployment, a rise in temporary employment, and unending layoffs in major industries: "We're in trouble right now because all our big industries are closing down. . . . We used to have a fairly stable and high-income working [population]. Blue-collar people populated all these neighborhoods around here, and they could make good money at Bethlehem Steel and other factories around, and so we're slipping. We're slipping because we're losing that big industry

and we're not attracting anything else. I think we're slipping economically" (Nancy Moore). These changes and the misery they produced
in turn were often perceived to be connected to a shift from a primarily industrial economy to a service economy: "In Baltimore, I see
the group that has the wealth moving ahead more rapidly than the
group that does not have the wealth. So I see the split happening faster,
and I also see the group at the bottom in Baltimore growing much
faster than I do somewhere else. Everybody talks about the change
from industrial economy to a service economy, I think that's a very real
thing. . . . But it's broader than that too, because there's a lot of preju-
dice involved" (Eliot Green).

Many people to whom we talked experienced these large-scale economic transformations within the life spans of their own parents and
siblings:

> Well, I figure Baltimore's probably a blue-collar town, from after
> World War II up till . . . the late seventies, early eighties, but dur-
> ing that time, industry started to decline, you saw the GM plant
> like close down, Bethlehem Steel really took a dive, Martin
> Marietta cut back on who they employed. [In the] early seven-
> ties, that's when they started redoing the Inner Harbor, and they
> became more of a service-oriented type of industry. Downtown
> Baltimore is tourism now, and I mean nobody would have dreamt
> that twenty-five, thirty years ago. And now it's more professional
> or white-collar type of jobs than I can remember growing up; my
> dad worked for the railroad, the B&O. . . . And now I don't know
> of that many people that work in industry that much any more. I
> mean they're office workers or, you know, the professionals.
> (Barbara McGuire)

The rest of this book describes many facets of an emerging worldview in the United States in the late twentieth century, a worldview
that encompasses notions about how persons, bodies, and organizations
are put together and how they function in health or illness. The dramatic changes in social and economic organization that we just heard
several people describe are part of the overall context out of which this
worldview is emerging. My task is to describe this emerging worldview
in relation to many different ideas, from scientific knowledge about the
body to management theories about organizations. To avoid any mis-

understanding, I should state up front, however, that I do not ettempt
to determine priority or causation, to determine which notion or phenomenon came first and caused another to come into being or influenced its development in some way. That task demands too fine a level
of discrimination for a set of phenomena too massively overdeter-
mined. It also demands too definitive a notion of causality to capture
the sundry and dissimilar beliefs and actions that are emerging in various elusive relationships with each other.

PART THREE

VISIONS OF THE
IMMUNE SYSTEM

IN THE FOLLOWING SECTION, I DESCRIBE HOW THE EMERGING entity, the immune system, looks from various points of view in our society. Since the substantive issues that concern me relate to the status of scientific knowledge, what scientists have to say makes up one chapter. But I have juxtaposed what scientists say to what is said by those in several other positions: the media; people who are not scientific or medical experts; people who define themselves as experts in some form of alternative medicine.

In my previous work, I tried to identify differences in worldview that might go along with differences in social position determined by factors such as gender, age, or class. Here, the reader should be forewarned, I am engaged in a different enterprise. This is not to say that the kinds of differences that I identified in my earlier work are unimportant or that for another purpose at another time I would not choose to draw them out. But my goal here is to describe an emerging sensibility quite different from that of the recent past. The main problematic, then, is how widespread is this sensibility? Will people in widely separated social positions articulate some version of it?

CHAPTER 1

The Body at War: Media Views of the Immune System

But the thing that sticks to my mind more than anything else is, do you remember the movie The Fantastic Voyage? *Where they shoved people down inside the body? Do you remember the scene when they had to go outside the ship to fix the cell, and the little antibodies were coming all around them and everything like that? I think that's where I get a lot of my ideas from, you know? That was probably the first real exposure I had to the human body and the immune system, because I was young, I was still in elementary school.*

CHARLES KINGSLEY

When Mack Drury found out that his lover had tested HIV+, he told us, he faced the difficult task of getting himself tested. At the clinic he visited, Mack and the others in the waiting room watched a film about AIDS that illustrated graphically how HIV will destroy the cells in your immune system. He said that he fled from the clinic, disturbed because the images and language in the film were so upsetting, and afraid that his health would be affected by them.

Mack's conviction that his health would be harmed by the images in the film made me want to explore in some detail media coverage of the immune system. I include here audio, print, and other visual media that are usually available to a mass audience. I do not include technical publications in the sciences because I will deal with them in Chapter 4.

Perhaps the notion of an immune "system" was first widely disseminated to the reading public through an article condensed in the *Reader's Digest* in 1957 (Brecher and Brecher 1957). Accompanying a small but steady rate of publications about the immune system in mass market magazines throughout the 1960s and 1970s, two major film productions featured the immune system.[1] *The Fantastic Voyage*, starring Raquel Welch, first appeared in 1966, and several people we interviewed mentioned that they remembered it vividly. (It is now available in local video stores.) Several main components of the immune system (antibodies, macrophages, lymph nodes) had a role to play in the film, which involved miniaturizing a submarine for travel through the arteries and veins of a Russian scientist who had defected from the Soviet Union. The scientist had been so severely injured that conventional surgery would have been no use. The goal of the crew was to remove a blood clot caused by his injury so the Russian could recover consciousness and divulge Soviet secrets to the Americans. The team of medical specialists and army personnel inside the submarine tried to travel through the Russian's body to reach the site of his injury, which they attempted to repair with a laser. Along the way, caught while wearing a diving suit outside the submarine, Raquel Welch was attacked by antibodies. These were depicted as flickering shapes that adhered tightly to her chest and nearly suffocated her, until, just in the nick of time, the male members of the team managed (more than slightly lasciviously) to pull them off with their hands. In the end, the villain of the drama (a double agent) was horribly killed, suffocated by the billowing white mass of a macrophage as the ship passed through a lymph node.

In the early 1970s, a television program called "The Immortal" featured a hero who had a "supercharged immune system that made him impervious to the diseases and the gradual wearing down the flesh is heir to. Traumas like a bullet to the heart could kill the guy, but if he survived, his wounds would heal within hours" (Laliberte 1992:56; see also Terrace 1985–86:215).

Riding the crest of the huge wave of media interest in the immune system that began in the early 1980s, science writers such as Peter Jaret published major articles on the immune system and embellished them with electron micrographs of immune system cells and their interactions. According to the readers' survey carried out by the National

Geographic Society, Jaret's 1986 photographic essay garnered the most commendations of any article published that year and prompted a large number of requests for reprints.[2]

Jaret's essay in the *National Geographic* apparently inspired writers for several other mass media periodicals, which shortly thereafter featured cover stories on the immune system (see figs. 7, 8): *Time* (Jaroff 1988), *U.S. News and World Report* (Brownlee 1990), and *Awake!* (November 1990).[3] The *Reader's Digest* once again presented a major article on the immune system, this time a condensation of Jaret's article (Jaret 1987).

At the same time, the syndrome that we now call AIDS was beginning to be understood as an immune system dysfunction, enormously increasing both scientific and public interest in how the immune system works or fails to work. Beginning in the early 1980s, there was an explosion of interest in periodicals on the immune system, whether measured in absolute numbers or as a percentage of all articles in periodicals.[4] Apart from periodicals, other print media on the immune system mushroomed. Here I can give only the slightest indication of the quantity of this material by indicating its range. There are books that combine science education with practical guidelines for a healthy immune system (e.g., Dwyer 1988; Fox and Fox 1990; Pearsall 1987; Potts and Morra 1986). There are books that appeal to methods of strengthening the immune system that are intended to be different from those of biomedicine (e.g., Chopra 1989; DeSchepper 1989; Michaud and Feinstein 1989; Muramoto 1988; Serinus 1987). There is also a special genre of children's books on the immune system (e.g., Benziger 1989, 1990; Galland 1988; Gelman 1992).

As one would expect given the flourishing of books and magazines, there are many audiotapes devoted to the health of the immune system, subliminal and otherwise (e.g., Sutphen 1988; Mars 1992; Achterberg and Lawlis 1992). There are also high school and college science teaching films galore (*The Human Immune System: The Fighting Edge, Immune System Disorders, Lupus,* and *Internal Defenses* are examples from one catalog),[5] science films for grade school and middle school students (*The Immune System: Your Magic Doctor, The Immune System: Our Internal Defender*),[6] seminars for health professionals of all sorts,[7] and seminars for continuing adult education.[8]

The portrait of the body conveyed most often and most vividly in the mass media shows it as a defended nation-state, organized around

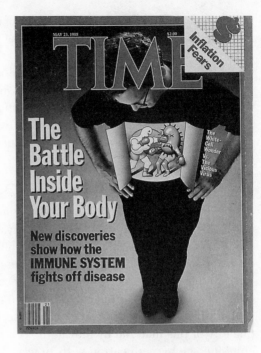

Fig. 7. *The body's immune system (the white-cell wonder) shown in a boxing match with the vicious virus. From* Time, *23 May 1988. © 1988 Time Inc. Reprinted by permission.*

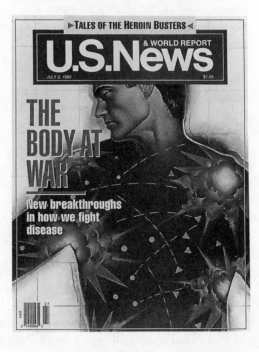

Fig. 8. *The body at war encapsulates* U.S. News and World Report's *cover story on the immune system. From* U.S. News and World Report, *2 July 1990. Reprinted with permission of the publisher.*

a hierarchy of gender, race, and class.[9] In this picture, the boundary between the body ("self") and the external world ("nonself") is rigid and absolute: "At the heart of the immune system is the ability to distinguish between self and nonself. Virtually every body cell carries distinctive molecules that identify it as self" (Schindler 1988:1). These molecules are class 1 MHC proteins, present on every nucleated cell in an individual's body and different from every other individual's. One popular book calls these our "trademark" (Dwyer 1988:37). The maintenance of the purity of self within the borders of the body is seen as tantamount to the maintenance of the self: a chapter called "The Body under Seige," in the popular book on the immune system *In Self Defense,* begins with an epigraph, from Shakespeare: "To be or not to be, that is the question" (Mizel and Jaret 1985:1).[10]

The notion that the immune system maintains a clear boundary between self and nonself is often accompanied by a conception of the nonself world as foreign and hostile.[11] Our bodies are faced with masses of cells bent on our destruction: "To fend off the threatening horde, the body has devised astonishingly intricate defenses" (Schindler 1988:13). As a measure of the extent of this threat, popular publications depict the body as the scene of total war between ruthless invaders and determined defenders:[12] "Besieged by a vast array of invisible enemies, the human body enlists a remarkably complex corps of internal bodyguards to battle the invaders" (Jaret 1986:702). A site of injury is "transformed into a battle field on which the body's armed forces, hurling themselves repeatedly at the encroaching microorganisms, crush and annihilate them" (Nilsson 1985:20).

Small white blood cells called *granulocytes* are "kept permanently at the ready for a blitzkrieg against microorganisms" and constitute the "infantry" of the immune system. "Multitudes fall in battle, and together with their vanquished foes, they form the pus which collects in wounds." Larger macrophages are another type of white blood cell that is depicted as the "armoured unit" of the defense system. "These roll forth through the tissues . . . devouring everything that has no useful role to play there." Another part of the immune system, the complement system, can "perforate hostile organisms so that their lives trickle to a halt." These function as " 'magnetic mines.' They are sucked toward the bacterium and perforate it, causing it to explode" (Nilsson 1985:24, 25, 24, 72). When complement "comes together in the right sequence, it detonates like a bomb, blasting through the invader's cell membrane" (Jaret 1986:720). The *killer cells*, the technical scientific name of a type of T lymphocyte, are the "immune system's special combat units in the war against cancer." Killer cells "strike," "attack," and "assault" (Nilsson 1985:96, 98, 100). "The killer T cells are relentless. Docking with infected cells, they shoot lethal proteins at the cell membrane. Holes form where the protein molecules hit, and the cell, dying, leaks out its insides" (Jaroff 1988:59).

To understand the immune system, we are to think of it "as a disciplined and effective army that posts soldiers and scouts on permanent duty throughout your body" (Laliberte 1992:56). These warriors identify a threat, attack and destroy our enemies so quickly that we often do not know that we were threatened: the immune system "never takes prisoners." The story of the human immune system "reads like a war novel": our lymph nodes are major centers for the breeding of "attack dogs," called antibodies (Gates 1989:16). In sum, the body "has devised a series of defenses so intricate they make war games look like child's play" (National Institute of Allergy and Infectious Diseases 1985:5).

Although the metaphor of warfare against an external enemy dominates these accounts, another metaphor plays nearly as large a role: the body as police state.[13] Every body cell is equipped with "'proof of identity' — a special arrangement of protein molecules on the exterior . . . these constitute the cell's identity papers, protecting it against the body's own police force, the immune system. . . . The human body's police corps is programmed to distinguish between bona fide residents and illegal aliens — an ability fundamental to the body's powers of self-defence" (Nilsson 1985:21). What identifies a resident is likened to speaking a national language: "An immune cell bumps into a bacterial cell and says, 'Hey, this guy isn't speaking our language, he's an intruder.' That's defense" (Levy, quoted in Jaret 1986:733). "T cells are able to 'remember for decades' the identity of foreign antigens: the intruders' descriptions are stored in the vast criminal records of the immune system. When a substance matching one of the stored descriptions makes a new appearance, the memory cells see to the swift manufacture of antibodies to combat it. The invasion is defeated before it can make us ill. We are *immune*" (Nilsson 1985:28).

What happens to these illegal aliens when they are detected? They are "executed" in a "death cell," the digestive cavity inside a feeding cell (Nilsson 1985:25, 31, 76, 81). "When the walls have closed around the enemy, the execution — phagocytosis — takes place. The prisoner is showered with hydrogen peroxide or other deadly toxins. Digestive enzymes are sent into the death chamber to dissolve the bacterium" (Nilsson 1985:81).

Not surprisingly, identities involving gender, race, and class are present in this war scene. Compare two categories of immune system cells, macrophages, which surround and digest foreign organisms, on the one hand, and T cells, which kill by transferring toxin to them, on the other. The macrophages are a lower form of cell; they are called a "primeval tank corps" (Michaud and Feinstein 1989:4), "a nightmare lurching to life" (Page 1981:115). T cells are more advanced, evolutionarily, and have higher functions, such as memory (Jaroff 1988:60). It is only these advanced cells who "attend the technical colleges of the immune system" (Nilsson 1985:26).

There is clearly a hierarchical division of labor here, one that is to some extent overlaid with gender categories familiar in European and American culture. Specifically, one might wonder about the female associations with the engulfing and surrounding that macrophages do and the male associations with the penetrating or injecting that killer T cells do. In addition, many scholars have pointed out the frequent association of the female, symbolically, with lower functions, especially with the lack or lesser degree of mental functions.

Beyond this, macrophages are the cells that are the "housekeepers" (Jaret 1986) of the body, cleaning up the dirt and debris, including "dead bodies," both themselves and foreign cells. (One immunologist called them "little drudges.")[14] "The first defenders to arrive would be the phagocytes [a category of 'eating' cells that includes macrophages] — the scavengers of the system. Phagocytes constantly scour the territories of our bodies, alert to anything that seems out of place. What they find, they engulf and consume. Phagocytes are not choosy. They will eat anything suspicious that, they find in the bloodstream, tissues, or lymphatic system" (Jaret 1986:715). Given their uncultivated origins, it should not be surprising that, after eating, a macrophage "burps": "After it finishes its meal, it burps out pieces of the enemy and puts them out on its surface" (Michaud and Feinstein 1989:6). As macrophages feed, they may be described as "angry," in a "feeding fury," or "insatiable" (Page 1981:104), combining in one image uncontrolled emotions and an obliterating, engulfing presence, both common cultural ascriptions of females.

Gender might not be the only overlay on the division of labor in our cells. Racial overtones may be there as well, although I have less convincing evidence for them. Macrophages are the cells that actually eat other cells belonging to the category *self* and so engage in "a kind of small-scale cannibalism" (Nilsson 1985:25). Cannibalism is often associated with the attribution of a lower, animal nature to those who engage in it (Arens 1979). In media coverage of the immune system, macrophages are seen as feminized in some ways but as simply "uncivilized" in others. These "cannibals" are indiscriminate eaters, barbaric and savage in their willingness to eat any manner of thing at all. Sometimes macrophages are feminized "housekeepers," and sometimes they seem to be marked by race, class, or a combination of the two, as when they are described as "big, primitive garbage collectors" (Jaret 1986:733), "roving garbage collectors" (Brownlee 1990:50), a "'cleanup' crew" (Pearsall 1987:41), or "roving scavengers" (Jaroff 1988:58).

To explore further the popular media imagery of the hierarchy of cells, we need to look at another immune system cell, the B cell. B cells are clearly ranked far above the lowly macrophage. They are not educated in the college of the thymus, but they are "educated" in the bone marrow (Dwyer 1988:47), and they have enormous specificity. They rank below the T cell, however, which is consistently termed the *orchestrator* of the immune response and which activates B cells. In one popular book, this is called giving the B cell "permission" (Dwyer 1988:47) to attack invading organisms. B cells exist in two stages, immature and mature B cells. Mature B cells are the cells that, having been stimulated by antigens of the right specificity, and with T cell "permission," rapidly produce antibodies against invading antigens. In a children's book about the immune system, all the immune system cells are given names and identities. The B cell, called "Bubbles" (see fig. 9), bulged "big and bright" as she began to make antibodies. When "Major D," a type of T cell, gives the order, "Bubbles danced about as she emptied bag after bag into the blood" (Benziger 1990:20).

This suggests that B cells are sometimes feminized but rank much higher in the hierarchy than the lowly macrophage.[15] This means that in the B cell we may have a kind of upper-class female, a suitable partner for the top-ranked T cell. These two types of cells together have been termed "the mind of the immune system" (Galland 1988:10). In illustrations of these cells in *Peak Immunity* (see fig. 10), each of them is depicted with a drawing of a human brain (DeSchepper 1989:16). Far below them in terms of class and race we would find the macrophage, angry and engulfing, or scavenging and cleaning up.

In this system, gendered distinctions are not limited to male and female; they also encompass the distinction between heterosexual and homosexual. T cells convey aspects of male potency, cast as heterosexual potency. They are the virile heroes of the immune system, highly trained commandos who are selected for and then educated in the technical college of the thymus gland. T cells are referred to as the "commander in chief of the immune system" (Jaret 1986:708) or the "battle manager" (Jaroff 1988:58). Some T cells, killer cells, are masculine in the old-fashioned mold of a brawny, brutal he-man: in a mail advertisement from *Prevention* magazine for a book (i.e., Michaud and Feinstein 1989) on the immune system, we are told, "You owe your life to this little guy, the Rambo of your body's immune system." A comic book produced for AIDS education depicts T cells as a squad of Mister

Fig. 9. *A depiction of a B cell as "Bubbles," who is dancing about as she empties antibodies into the blood. From J. Benziger,* The Corpuscles: Adventure in InnerSpace *(1898:20). Reprinted with permission of the author.*

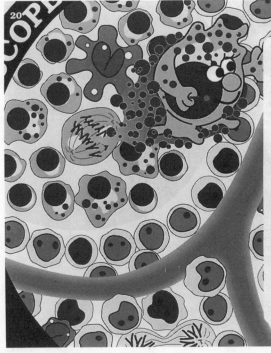

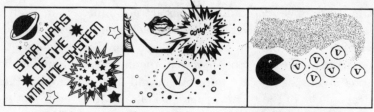

Virus attacks!

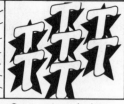

The body's phagocyte (the "Pac Man" of the immune system) attacks the viruses.

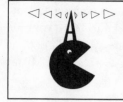

"Pac Man" displaying the antigen.

The "Pac Man" displaying the antigen alerts the T-Helper cell. (Commander-in-chief of our immune

Once activated, the T-Helper cells begin to multiply.

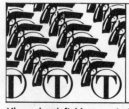

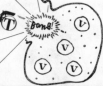

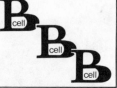

Like a battlefield general, the T-Helper cells send for the front soldiers called T-Killer cells!

They puncture membranes of the infected cells, disrupting the cycle of the viruses.

The T-Helper cells then call in the second platoon called B-Cells!

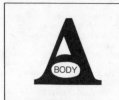

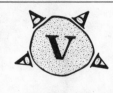

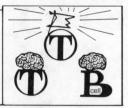

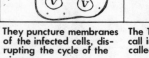

The B-Cells produce chemical weapons called antibodies.

Antibodies not only neutralize, but kill.

A truce is signed by the T-Suppressor. T and B-Memory cells are left in our body.

Fig. 10. *Star wars of the immune system, showing T cells and B cells with brains and memory. From L. DeSchepper,* Peak Immunity *(1989:15–16). Reprinted with permission of the author.*

Ts, (see fig. 11), the muscular hero from the television show "The A Team."

Other T cells, T 4 cells, have a masculinity composed of intellect, strategic planning ability, and a propensity for corporate team partici- pation, powers well suited for the world of global corporations.[16] The T 4 cell is often called *the quarterback of the immune system* because he orchestrates everything else and because he is the brains and memory of the team. As one source puts it, "Besides killer T cells . . . there are also helper [T 4] and suppressor T cells. *Somebody* has to make strate- gic decisions." This popular manual on the immune system, called *Fighting Disease*, clinches the heterosexuality of the T cell: "In order to slip inside a cell, a virus has to remove its protein coat, which it leaves outside on the cell membrane. The viral coat hanging outside signals the passing T cell that viral hanky panky is going on inside. Like the jealous husband who spots a strange jacket in the hall closet and *knows* what's going on in the upstairs bedroom, the T cell takes swift action. It bumps against the body cell with the virus inside and perforates it" (Michaud and Feinstein 1989:10, 8).

However they are marked by gender, sexuality, race, or class, all these cells of the immune system belong to "self" and have the primary function of defending the self against the nonself. When the nonself is a disease-causing microbe, the model works quite logically. But when the nonself is a fetus growing inside a woman's body, the model quickly runs into difficulty. As the popular media explain it, since the fetus is a graft of foreign tissue inside the mother, why does she not "mount an attack against the fetus as she would against any other allo- graft [a graft from a genetically different member of the same species]?" (Kimball 1986:433). The lack of an attack is even more mys- terious given that pregnant women have antibodies to certain antigens expressed by the fetus. The reduction in the woman's normal immune response, which would be to destroy the fetal "nonself," whatever the mechanism, is called *tolerance*. From an immunological point of view, the fetus is a "tumor" that the woman's body should try furiously to attack (Dwyer 1988:60). But the mother's immune system "tolerates" her fetus; all our immune systems "tolerate" our own tissues, unless we suffer from autoimmune disease.

Immunologists have yet fully to answer the question of how the body achieves tolerance; in the meantime, it is interesting to wonder whether other images of the body less reliant on hard boundaries and strict distinctions might produce another set of questions altogether.

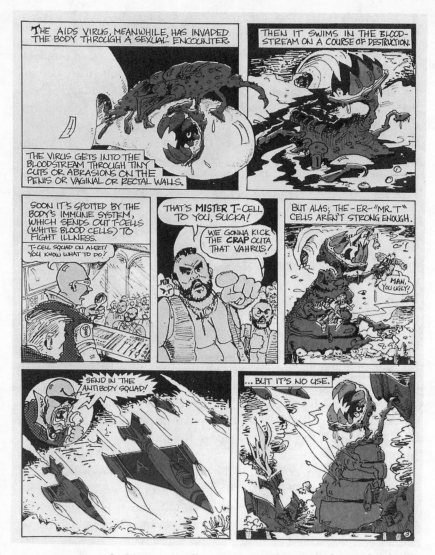

Fig. 11. *A squad of Mister T cells attempts to do in HIV but is defeated. From D. Cherry, "AIDS Virus," in* Risky Business *(1988:5). Reprinted with permission of the publisher. Credit San Francisco AIDS Foundation.*

Work in feminist theory suggests that there is a masculinist bias to views that divide the world into sharply opposed, hostile categories, such that the options are to conquer, be conquered, or magnanimously tolerate the other. The stance is one from which nature can be dominated and a separation from the world maintained (Keller 1985:124).[17] Many mothers and fathers might find the notion of a baby in utero as a tumor that the mother's body tries its best to destroy so counterintuitive as to warrant searching for a different set of organizing images altogether.[18]

Another set of images coexists in the popular media with these scenes of battle and is also imbued with hierarchies involving gender and class. This other set of images coexists uneasily with the first, is subdued by taking up far less space in printed descriptions, and is able to generate far fewer visual images to express itself. It depicts the body as a "regulatory-communications network" (Schindler 1988:1). As Haraway's work emphasizes, the body is seen as "an engineered communications system, ordered by a fluid and dispersed command-control-intelligence network" (1989:14). Hierarchy is replaced by dispersed control; rigidly prescribed roles are replaced by rapid change and flexible adaptation. The emphasis shifts from the various roles played by the parts of the immune system to "the most remarkable feature of the immune system . . . the system itself — the functioning of diverse elements as an efficient, effective whole" (National Jewish Center for Immunology and Respiratory Medicine 1989:2). As an example, consider a pamphlet on the immune system that is available from the National Cancer Institute.[19] In the midst of elaborate military metaphors —"defense against foreign invaders," "stockpiling a tremendous arsenal," "intricate defenses to fend off the threatening horde,"— a very different set of images appears: The immune system is described as "an incredibly elaborate and dynamic regulatory-communications network. Millions and millions of cells, organized into sets and subsets, pass information back and forth like clouds of bees swarming around a hive. The result is a sensitive system of checks and balances that produces an immune response that is prompt, appropriate, effective, and self-limiting" (Schindler 1988:1). This is an image of a complex system held together by communication and feedback, not divided by category and hierarchy. Often, in this mode, accounts stress how rapidly the system can be poised to change in response to its environment. Description of that process can easily slip back into the military analogy: "By storing just a few cells specific for each potential invader, it [the immune system] has room for the entire array. When an antigen appears, these few specifically matched cells are stimulated to multiply into a full-scale army. Later, to prevent this army from overexpanding wildly, like a cancer, powerful suppressor mechanisms come into play"

(National Institute of Allergy and Infectious Diseases 1985:3). One way in which a few accounts diminish the tension between these two images is specifically to stress the changed character of contemporary warfare: the great variety of different "weapons" is a product of evolutionary adaptation to changing defense needs: "Just as modern arsenals are ever changing as the weaponry of a potential enemy becomes more sophisticated, so our immune system has adapted itself many times to counter survival moves made by the microbial world to protect itself" (Dwyer 1988:28).

In sum, for the most part, the media coverage of the immune system operates largely in terms of the image of the body at war. Even when the problem is not an external enemy like a microbe but an internal part of "self," the military imagery is extended to notions of "mutiny," "self-destruction," and so on.[20] In one television show, autoimmunity was described as "we have met the enemy and the enemy is us."[21] A book on AIDS written by a physiologist for a general audience repeatedly refers to autoimmunity as "the immunological equivalent of civil war" (Root-Bernstein 1993:87) (for another example of autoimmune disease conceptualized as civil war, see fig. 12).[22]

Powerful as the impact of media images may be, we would be terribly misled if we took their content as the only sign of what is being understood in the wider culture. Many studies assume that the content of mass media products gives transparent evidence of "cultural ideas." Some further assert that the mass media do not allow any meaningful response from the public: they are "opposed to mediation"; they "fabricate noncommunication" (Baudrillard 1985).[23] Ethnographic exploration will quickly show us that the reality is far more complex. In the end, we will see that media images, rich as they seem, are impoverished in comparison to the living collage of ideas produced by people — scientists and nonscientists.

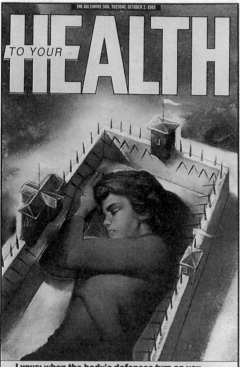

Fig. 12. *A woman with lupus shown inside her body's castle. Although the walls are thick and strong, the spikes of the castle's defenses are turned inward, threatening her. From the cover of* To Your Health, *3 October 1989. This illustration used courtesy of The Baltimore Sun Company. © 1993 The Baltimore Sun.*

CHAPTER 2

Immunology on the Street:
How Nonscientists See
the Immune System

> *They knew about the digestive system 'cause they had to eat, and*
> *they knew about the circulatory system because sometimes they*
> *bleed, by accidentally cutting themselves or falling. But who on*
> *earth has ever thought about the immune system? Only the elite few,*
> *people with allergies, understood, you know? Only the elite few, and*
> *now everybody else has got to learn about this thing? The immune*
> *system that's everywhere in the body? And, oh my God, what is a*
> *thymus gland?*
>
> JEWELL FRANKLIN

> *I mean the whole purpose of your studies is a sort of immunology*
> *on the street.*
>
> BRUCE KLEINER

Does "the immune system" live in the popular imagination?
When I began this study, I was quite prepared to have this
question answered negatively or at least indifferently. Although, as we
will see in more detail in Chapter 8, by the 1990s the immune system
had a robust existence in the disciplines of science, and although, as
we saw in the last chapter, it had made many dramatic appearances on
the stage of print and video media, these developments did not necessarily mean that ordinary people without training in the sciences
would have much to say on the subject.

As we began to have conversations and carry out extended interviews in several neighborhoods, it quickly became apparent that peo-

ple had a great deal to say about the immune system. The topic itself, set in the context of a general discussion about health and well-being, seemed to open up an imaginative field in which people readily explored their ideas about the body and society.

What became clear is that the media coverage of the immune system, as seen in the last chapter, does not encompass very well the body imagery with which people are in fact operating. The dominant message of the media, clothed in the accoutrements of warfare, accompanied by the trappings of the hierarchies of gender, race, and class, would be very misleading if we were to take it as evidence of how people are thinking. Other, subordinate messages present in the media, not as vividly brought to the fore — depictions of complex, nonhierarchical systems embedded in environments composed of other complexly interacting systems — are what many people have already given a lively existence in their daily lives and commonsense conceptions. In a sense, the ground on which the old-style immune armies would march has already been seized by completely new forces, who have something other than war in mind.

THE BASIC IDEA

In our interviews, the most fundamental, widespread agreement — across all social categories of age, gender, class, and sexuality — about the immune system is that it is something inside our bodies that protects us from disease. John Marcellino explains the shift in his thinking from germs that "just didn't come in" to "something inside that fights these things."

> *Suppose that you're with a person that has something that is contagious, say the flu. And you do not get the flu. What would you say is happening inside you at that point?*
> What's happening inside of you is that your body is somehow fighting off those germs. I saw a National Geographic video, they had this thing, I think it's in your white blood cells or something, and a germ would go into your body, and this thing would like surround it.
> *The white blood cell?*
> Yeah, and it would come around, and then it would eat it. And that's what happens. . . . I would say probably before what I thought happened is that you were just lucky not to get it, it

just didn't come in, you know, didn't get to you. But I understand now.

But you didn't analyze it farther.

No. . . . I would say probably it's because you were taking care of yourself. You know, you're getting enough sleep at night, you know what I mean, or you're eating good, or whatever. But now I understand that there's something inside your body that's fighting these things, and so these things come in, and they fight them off.

Echoes of the general idea that Marcellino expresses are exceedingly common in our interviews with people from every ethnic and socioeconomic background, every gender and generation. An African-American female teacher in her 40s told us: "Well, the immune system, I think, is that part of your body which fights off disease, and it's a very important part of your system. Without an immune system that's functioning properly, you're susceptible to pick up a lot of germs, diseases, etc." (Julia Sarton). When we asked "what the body does if you're around someone that's sick, and say you don't get sick," an elderly Euro-American male who was a retired seaman responded:

Well, I figure, what do they call them, you got, your immune. Your body builds up immunity to certain things, and if you're around a person has a certain type of sickness, if you don't get it, fine. . . .

So what's your understanding of how the immune system works?

It's something in your body. Something inside your body that blood builds up. And they got a lot of technical names I don't know, but they help you build up in your body immunity to these certain diseases. (Jack Morgan)

A Euro-American, male financial adviser in his twenties said:

I just know vague, vague things . . . basically that if your immune system works, it keeps you from being ill. If it doesn't work, you're susceptible to all kinds of things, whether it's the common cold or something like cancer or AIDS. I couldn't tell you where it's located.

*So can you sort of speculate on how the system actually
works or what's involved in the function?*
Well, I mean I know there are antibodies that fight intruding
bacteria or virus. I don't know if those things pop off the cell,
you know, and invade these viruses or what have you. And I
know that they have something to do with the white cells, I
think.
*But do you know how all these things work together?
What are the white blood cells doing, or, you mentioned
antibodies?*
Well, I think the white cells are killer cells, they kill off bacteria
and unwanted particles that get into the blood stream, I guess.
Red blood cells, I guess, keep you healthy otherwise. I don't
know. I hated science. (John Parker)

In spite of his assertion that he did not know where the immune system
is located, this interviewee, John Parker, offered to draw a picture of
his idea of the immune system, which shows how widely dispersed
throughout the body he imagines it to be (see fig. 13).

For most people, the system inside determines whether you are
going to get sick or stay well. As Sarah Christopher, a young African-
American fast-food worker, put it, in response to the question, "Well
tell me, let's say you've been hanging around someone who's sick, and
by all rules of nature you should have gotten sick too, but you don't
catch it. What do you think's protecting you? I mean why is it that you
don't have it?": "I must have antibodies, a strong immune system, just
fighting them off. . . . My immune system must go to say, you know,
you're not going to catch this, this is not for you to catch, and fight it
off, those little germs in the air." Katherine Johnson, a Euro-American
midwife in her thirties, explained how she would tell her son why she
caught a cold and he did not: "One way of looking at that is that I got
exposed to the bacteria and couldn't fight it and he could, and the other
way of looking at that is that we both got exposed, but my system didn't
hold up and his did. Or another way of looking at that is that we both
always had that bacteria, but because of stress or whatever, it was able
to take over in my system and not in his."

It seems to follow from a robust notion of an internal system of protection that the system exists to ward off continual threats. People focus
their attention on the well-being of the system rather than on creating
an environment that is free from threat. We have seen how the domi-

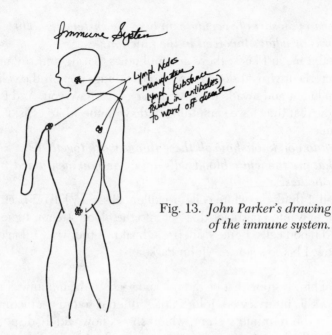

Fig. 13. *John Parker's drawing*
of the immune system.

nant model of disease prevention before 1970 focused on cleaning surfaces of the body and the house to keep them germ free. As we might
expect, people in our interviews frequently express the notion that the
environment surrounding our bodies contains many dangers that cannot ever be eliminated:

> *Why do you wipe the top of your soda can off?*
> Oh, because it's dirty, and it's germy, and I know even by wiping
> it, you noticed I used a wet cloth and then I dried it off? Even
> by wiping it, I'm still getting the germs, but at least I don't see
> that black dirt. I'm not putting my mouth up to it, but I know
> that it still gets dirty. I used to be really neurotic about certain
> things, like I wouldn't eat, I was just so, so fussy. If something
> dropped on the table, I wouldn't eat it cause it would, you
> know, probably get germs on it. Now I pick it up off the floor
> and eat it. I just know that I'm, you know, ingesting plenty of
> germs. I mean when you see the kitchens of some restaurants
> and stuff and it just grosses you out. (Gillian Lewis)

Nothing that I have said so far justifies my earlier claim that the
warfare model so common in the media does not provide the dominant

logic for these accounts of the immune system. In fact, there seems to be no dearth of military imagery used by the people we interviewed. For one man, an architect, the immune system is "an incredible policing thing, a system-wide authority that works" (Eliot Green). For a midwife, it is "a monitoring system and a defense system at the same time" (Katherine Johnson). For a special education teacher, the immune system is "like our army. We have the army and then we have special forces. . . . If one level of protection fails, the next step is taken. The body won't give up unless we give up" (Jewell Franklin). A reporter draws a picture (see fig. 14) to illustrate how it was "fascinating there was this little war going on in your body; the good cells are fighting the bad cells" (Joel Robertson). Laura Peterson comments that "the only thing modern medicine uses is this image of fighting, which is sort of a warlike image, so that's what I think I'll [draw]. I don't really know that that's accurate, but it's ingrained in my mind" (see fig. 15).

To put these uses of military metaphors in a more complicated context, we asked people to reflect specifically on their import. We did this while showing people media images of the body at war (covers of *Time* and *U.S. News and World Report* — see figs. 7 and 8 above). Given this opportunity, several people burst forth with statements about what they saw as the dire consequences of using militaristic imagery to picture what goes on inside the body. Peter Rodriguez, for example, thought that

> the military motif is an unhealthy way of constructing it because
> . . . it supports the military's kind of power structure and sexism
> of society. . . . I think another effect of this military conception of

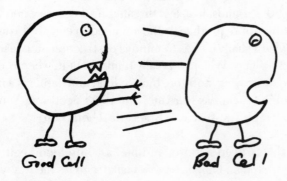

Fig. 14. *Joel Robertson's drawing of the immune system.*

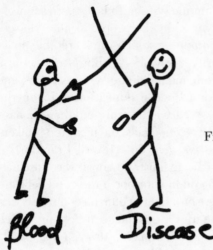

Fig. 15. *Laura Peterson's drawing
of the immune system.*

the whole thing is it puts the conception into that of a foreign invasion, and there's this outsider that we don't like who's in our midst, and we want them to get out, and we have to resort to violence to get rid of them. I think that only sparks violence against people. I think that only supports everyone's homophobia. I think it only supports everybody's xenophobia.

Although most people did not have such well-formulated positions, many were able to produce a plethora of alternative images, such as eating (Brackette Thompson), dancing or playing (Sarah Christopher), or simply convincing it to go away (David Feldman):

The whole thing of war is not one that I take to very well. I mean, eating, this sounds, like, less threatening, because when you think of eating you're just like, "Oh, you need to eat." But you think of war, what usually comes to mind is destruction and death and all of these things. When you really think about it, when you eat, like you're destroying stuff too, but . . . food and eating is a necessary part of life, whereas war isn't. You don't need war. You need to eat to, you know, survive. (Brackette Thompson)

See, this is Fred Astaire, and he's a white blood cell, and he's going to step on Ginger Rogers's head, and it's the way, you know, he does it. . . . Or make a game out of it. You're the white blood cell, and I'm the red blood cell. So, hey, that would be excellent, make a game out of it. You know, the white blood cell get the red blood cell, and we would box or, you know, play a game of charades or something. So I guess there are a lot of different ways of looking at it. (Sarah Christopher)

I've always thought of it as somehow eliminating it, rather than destroying it, and more subsuming it, depriving it of its power, more passive. Somehow less of a clash, more of a "convince it to go away" kind of thing. Show it the door rather than . . . somehow that seems more peaceful to me, that it takes it in and somehow digests the cell and then fits into the life cycle. Take the bad guys and use them for your own good rather than destroying them. (David Feldman)

There are many possible reasons why people would frequently choose a militaristic image first but, when offered the chance, could come up with many different images. The omnipresence of military imagery in the media and the authority carried by information about a scientific topic are possible relevant factors. But the kind of society and world in which different people grow up may also be important. In our interviews, all manner of people could produce military images: young people, old people, and especially aging baby boomers, who came of age during the cold war era of the 1940s and 1950s, when imagery of the body as a fortress or a castle was most vibrant. But *all* the examples that struck me as the most elaborated, vivid departures from military imagery came from people in their late teens and early twenties, people coming of age at a time when cold war assumptions are being drastically shaken and a new sensibility about how the body relates to the world may be arising.

In spite of my assertion that complex notions of the immune system occur throughout the interviews, there were a few cases in which someone had absolutely nothing to say on the subject. These instances include a teenage single mother who was unemployed, a couple in their seventies whose models of the body fit very well with the pre-1970 models discussed in Chapter 3, and a social worker in her forties. I could understand the relative isolation of the young mother and the older couple, but the social worker's response remained a puzzle until she happened to mention that she was legally blind and so never read newspapers or magazines and never watched television. In a real sense, these are exceptions that prove the rule. Being isolated from public culture — for whatever reason — may be the only way to escape acquiring, relating to, and worrying about an immune system.

Another way in which to see the complexity of people's thinking about health and their bodies is to look in some detail at how people have developed ways of looking at the immune system as a *complex system*. While I will undertake a more thorough analysis of what a complex system is and what it entails in Chapter 10, my goal here is simply to show how the basic elements of this idea permeate the accounts that people gave us of how their bodies work.

Two accounts that include most of the main elements of the way in which the immune system is often thought to work are these:

> Basically, it's a real complicated series of things that ties everything together. And when something goes wrong in your body, signals go out, and cells go to attack it. I guess it's basically just a system of checks and balances, and most things the immune system in the body can deal with on its own. . . . For the most part, it just sort of keeps everything in line with the metabolic computer.
> *Metabolic computer — that's great! I love it!*[1]
> I guess it says, "You need some of this. You need some of this." This constantly controlling your body. Keep the good things running correctly and get rid of the bad things. (Arthur Harrison)

> What I learned was that the AIDS virus somehow hides in the body and the T cell doesn't know that it's there. And I thought, well, that makes sense. If we could find a way to expose it, then maybe the immune system, which is so complex and so intricate, beyond my wildest dreams, or a connecting network of things, could win. And I know my peers that have had AIDS, and I've spoken with them, they said, I would rather have been told I had cancer, 'cause at least they could have cut it out. . . . AIDS seems so massive. We all learn quickly when we get it or if we come close to someone, that the immune system goes from your fingertips to the end of your hair. I mean, it's everywhere in your body; you cannot get away from it. (Jewell Franklin)

Let us unpack the main elements of the way in which this system works. First, this system is not localized in particular places in the body. As Jewell Franklin says, "It's everywhere." Two men in their seventies (Jack Smith and John Braun) discussed *Time* magazine's illustration of the immune system as the white blood cell in a boxing match with the vicious virus. John Braun asserted that "the immune system is the whole body; it's not just the lungs or abdomen. . . . If I cut myself, doesn't my immune system start to work right away to prevent infection? So it's in your finger; I mean it's everywhere. So that would be my criticism to *Time* magazine."

This system is composed of a great many parts "beyond our wildest dreams." There *are* parts, and each has a job to do, but the point that interviewees stressed is that the parts work together in complex ways to make a whole: it is "a complete network, a backup system" (Peter Black). Some of the most vivid descriptions of this feature of the system came when we showed people the media illustrations of the immune system:

> *What do you think of their [*Time *magazine's] representation of the immune system? Does it make a lot of sense to you or no? Would you make it different?*
> Yeah, I would, you know, 'cause it's like I said, I don't think of the immune system as being a one-being thing. You know, I mean I would have a battle scene here, you know. Not just a fight, I would have a whole battle scene, kind of *Gone-with-the-Wind*-ish. (Charles Kingsley)

> *Is there anything that compares itself to the immune system? I mean, putting platelets and blood aside, if you had to pick something else that it reminds you of?*
> Fish. You ever seen the little cartoon where the bigger fish eats the little fish?
> *Sure.*
> And then the bigger fish eats the medium fish. It's kind of like that. But sometimes, the only problem is if the disease is as big as the other fish, as your immune system, that's when you have problems.
> *OK, so this is* Time *magazine. This, is this how you imagine the immune system to be?*

. . . Well, I think there's more than your white blood cells fighting. That's just totally too narrow. See, my fish was the whole system; it wouldn't just be the white blood cells. 'Cause you got all kinds of things. (Charlene Kelsey)

This is from a Time *magazine cover.*
"White cell wonder versus the virus, vicious virus." That could be a healthy person. . . . I'd want my white blood cells to be that healthy. Kind of like it makes you wonder why he's just watching instead of helping.
The man in the picture?
Yeah, instead of doing more to help.
Like what kind of thing?
Maybe show him taking some medicine or eating something healthy or something like that. What gets the white blood cell to be healthy, healthy enough to fight off the virus? (Tara Holcolm)

Charles imagines a panoramic view of a monumental battle scene in *Gone with the Wind*; Charlene imagines fish swallowing fish in an infinite regression to represent "the whole thing"; Tara imagines the person's daily activities intrinsically related to what the cells inside the body are doing.

Even though the immune system is "everywhere," it is clearly thought to interact with other complex systems in the body. Barbara McGuire develops a complex picture of how her uncle's cancer interfered with one system after another in his body. Finally, it even entered the management system in his brain. She commented that, when one system succumbs to cancer, it is hard for the others to maintain themselves because they are interdependent. Later in the interview, she sketched in imagination, and in an actual drawing (see fig. 16), her conception of how the parts of the body's immune system work together:

See, I think this is your body, and then you've got all these little critters that hang out in here, and they're guards. And when they see somebody trying to come in and hurt you, they'll go down, and they try to defend this. But, in order to have guards, these guys got to get fed someplace and get clothes. Your blood brings them stuff to make them like strong. . . . They got to get some kind of nurture or something to take care of themselves so they

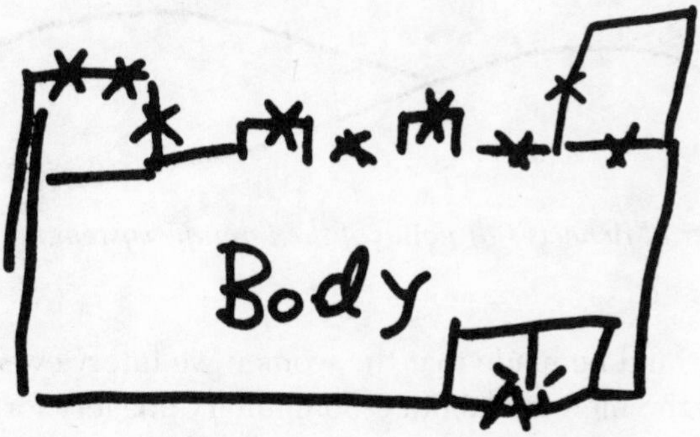

Fig. 16. *Barbara McGuire's drawing of the immune system.*

can take care of something coming into the door that you don't
want. They could have their own nice little sitting rooms. . . . Let's
say it's a normal house and you've got a leak in the roof. You
know, mom and dad go up to fix it. If you didn't feed mom or dad,
put some clothes on them, they couldn't do that. These little guys,
they've got a nice condo with a hot tub. (Barbara McGuire)

Even though she draws a picture of a fortress, stressing the older, pre-
1970s vision of the body's separation from the outside, what is added
here is the stress on the interdependence of its residents: the defending cells have to be cared for themselves in order to care for the body.

Vera Michaels objected to the *Time* cover because it depicts "such
violence going on in our bodies." She insisted that such violence is "not
in there." She claimed that her own representation would be "less dramatic":

My visualization would be much more like a piece of almost
tides or something . . . the forces, you know, the ebbs and flows.
Could you draw anything like that?
I could. I don't think anybody would perceive it as a portrayal
of the battle within.
What is it that ebbs and flows?
The two forces, I mean, the forces . . . imbalance and
balance.

As she spoke, she drew an illustration (see fig. 17), labeling it *the
waves*.

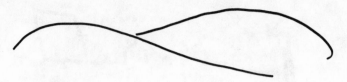

Fig. 17. *Vera Michaels's drawing of the immune system.*

A case could be made that the women we interviewed were more likely than the men to elaborate nonmilitary imagery for the immune system or to reject media images framed in those terms. In addition to the women I quote above, for example, Linda Rosen found "the whole battle notion and the boxing gloves and all that stuff . . . alienating. I don't feel like that's what happens inside my body. And I feel like it's a real male image of how the immune system works." But such a summary would not do justice to what we found. Not all women dislike military imagery, and some men reject it altogether. Among people we will meet later, a military veteran told us that his experiences fighting in Vietnam taught him that in war, as in the body's struggle for health, there is no way to know who the good guys are, and medical researchers have developed some astoundingly elaborate nonmilitary metaphors to describe the immune system. So there is no simple, linear, causal relation between one's identity as male or female and how one imagines the immune system. As we will see, this may have to do with some profound shifts that are taking place in the nature of identity itself.

In an article about the immune system, Donna Haraway asks, "Is there a way to turn the [military] discourse [of immunology] into an oppositional/alternative/liberatory approach? Is this postmodern body . . . *necessarily* an automated Star Wars battlefield in the now extraterrestrial space of the late twentieth-century Western scientific body's intimate interior?" (Haraway 1991:220–21). Among others, Vera Michaels, with her development of an image of ocean waves, tides ebbing and flowing in constant, turbulent change, begins to show us some possibilities.

So far, we have seen the immune system in popular imagination emerging as a complex, dispersed system intricately related to other complex systems. The relation between various systems is "flat" in the sense that no one is obviously in charge; different systems may play the most important role at different times. Jewell Franklin put it particularly vividly, again in response to the *Time* magazine illustration of the boxing cells. We enter the interview as she begins to draw her rendition of the immune system (see fig. 18).

> Well, this is my Neanderthal man.
> *OK.*
> OK? And we're going to make him happy because he doesn't have any diseases.
> *OK, great.*
> And one of the central points is in the chest bone. So I'm going to make that blue. It's going to happen right back here. And that's the thymus gland. And from that, this is where the T cells come. And there's this huge network that goes through the whole body. . . . And there's little glands over here, of course it's going to run into this person's brain, because the immune system is also, the endocrinology of the brain. . . . And there's this major network system that goes on. From that, though, you also have to consider the skeletal system. So now I want you to superimpose the skeletal system. And then of course we're going to have the bones, and this is going to be the knee joint, to the amphibia, or whatever those bones are. Inside the marrow of the bone, white cells, blood cells, are produced. This is necessary for the production of blood. This is important because if the thymus gland is affected in any way, then the T cells don't mature. . . . And the immune system is weakened. Now that I involved the bones, where the production is, you also have to include the circulatory system because that's how everything travels.

In line with the shifting nature of the roles played by different systems, the elements of the immune system are understood to operate in a nonlinear fashion. That is to say that elements of the system vary over time that and their ideal state at any one time may not be their ideal state at another. This is completely unlike linear variables such as strength or wealth, in which (perhaps) the more you have, the better off you are. When it comes to the immune system, many people think that the desirable amount of each substance or activity depends entirely on the total context. Too much of something can be as bad as too little.

This feature of the immune system was often stressed in our interviews in the many remarks people made about health problems that

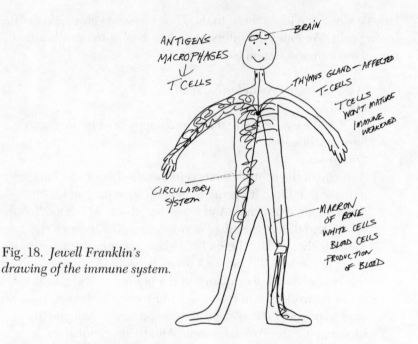

Fig. 18. *Jewell Franklin's*
drawing of the immune system.

they attributed to overly sensitive immune systems. To continue with
Jewell Franklin's narrative:

> *Here's an artist at* Time *magazine, the representation they've*
> *decided to use for the immune system. Does the way they*
> *depicted it make sense to you?*
> It makes sense to me. I think it's rather infantile, I think my
> explanation was better. [Laughs.] You know why? Because, at
> least to me, it leaves everybody hanging, you know. Well where
> did this white cell wonder come from? What's responsible for
> that? How do we promote more of it if it's so necessary, and do
> people even understand that if there's too much of it, that we
> have another disease. Too many white blood cells is not good.
> So people might think, Oh gee, if I go out and get some white
> blood cells, then I can fight viruses. Where can I buy them? I
> mean, we have a mentality like that out there.

To work effectively, a nonlinear system must be in constant change.
Like Jewell Franklin, other people talk about how elements of the
immune system increase or decrease (Joan Breslau), about how the
defenses of the body must be variable to deal with the many types of

viruses, which leads to the "tremendous effort required to keep me in equilibrium" (Brian Torok). Gillian Lewis explains how she sees the various components of the immune system changing over time.

> I'll just say, when the white blood count is up, then there's a virus. That's about all I know. . . . And there's a T helper and a T suppressor. And they've got to be healthy and suppressing something. I guess it must be the white blood cells, and like maybe there's too many T suppressor cells, so that makes the white blood count go down, and that's why there's not enough white blood cells to fight off disease. You have a lower blood count, white blood count, when you have HIV. You're not capable of fighting off viruses, you know, like most people can.

One of the most striking images of the immune system in change is that of a perpetual motion machine: "When I think about it in my head, I think of, you know, amoeba-like shapes moving through the body, being helpful when there's an issue or a crisis, or a contact point that's weakened, or something like that. And I think that's constant. For me I guess the best thing would be the perpetual motion machines. They always say that you can't invent a perpetual motion machine, but really, until we die, the bodies kind of are. That's what I think of it; I think of movement" (Wendy Marshall).

In what kind of change are these fluctuating mechanisms engaged? They are producing the different, specific things that the system needs at different times to handle whatever challenges it meets. In one account, "White blood cells are just a sort of generic fighters of whatever foreign matter enters the body, and antibodies are specific for certain types of viruses that come in. It's like a lock and key type thing, where the antibody is only a certain size and shape and it has to find the right size and shape. It has to fit a certain type of virus, or it won't work" (Marsha Wilmslow).

In one imaginative description, that the body specifically designs different products is attributed to a team of engineers: "Now this is just my understanding, the way that it can identify foreign substance. Duplicate it, and then send it somewhere for processing, to say, OK, now how do we get rid of this? And then this team of engineers breaks in and says 'Oh, we can do this, we can do this, we can do this, we can do this. Oh great. OK, well let's build it and send it out there.' And then the new whatever it is that your body has created sends it, and it kills it" (Phillip Monroe). In these and many other ways, people stressed the ability of the immune system constantly to change what it is producing to respond in a precise way to the constantly changing challenges presented. People told us that T cells can handle the unknown, even chemicals produced in a laboratory (Franklin Lamont); that, to handle viruses that are changing all the time, the immune system draws on an "inventory of resistance" (Gary Sullivan); that the immune system is differentiated, specialized, and always changing (Sally Felton); that the immune system is "continuously active" (Stephen Mattson); that the immune system shapes its response to fit, building things up so that they fit perfectly (Daniel Crofton).

Although people may or may not give the proper scientific names to the various components of the immune system (as scientists understand it), they readily and vividly convey their sense that the immune system is a complex system in interaction with other complex systems inside the body, a system that changes constantly in order to produce the specific things necessary to meet every challenge.

It is plain how detailed and ingenious people's accounts of the immune system can be. But what the words alone cannot convey is the tone in which they are said. Are people bored and indifferent, describing something they see as mundane? Are they filled with distaste or wariness, describing something they see as sinister? Or are they excited and awed, describing something they see as marvelous? In most cases, people spoke about the immune system with at least energetic interest. Quite often people would remark that they "valued" or "respected" their immune system. A few times people came forth with extended expressions of the awe in which they held it:

> Just that, this is the immune system, and it helps you fight disease. . . . That to me is one of the miracles of life itself. . . . I become speechless when I think of things like that. (Phillip Monroe)

> To me, the body is so mysterious. I think that there's elegance to it, its solutions to problems, the fact that it compensates so well. But I don't pretend to understand the mechanics of how it works — how antibodies recognize foreign objects, how they detect them, how they shape themselves. I don't know how the antibodies shape themselves. You see these drawings in scien-

tific shows where the virus is like this, and [the antibodies] build up just so they fit just perfectly in there. (Daniel Crofton)

This is going to sound hokey and all, but it really does make me marvel at what God has done for humans in things like the immune system and antibodies and things like that. That we are able to fight off infections, and kick them out, and prevent them from ever being hazardous again to us, things like that. And then you think about how frail people are, I mean, in reality how frail they really are. How one little germ or one little microscopic organism can put an end to a life. So, like I said, it sounds hokey, but. . . .
Yeah, it is pretty amazing. Just the whole orchestration of things going on, you know. . . .
How everything works — to perfection. At least, for the most part. (George Miller)

George Miller is envisioning the possibility of (near) perfection for the immune system in the face of the frightening frailty of human life. I return to this theme in later chapters, when we are in a position to see how notions of the perfectibility of this complex system are being attached in a crucial way to the notion that some kinds of people are superior to others.

CHAPTER 3

"Fix My Head": How Alternative Practitioners See the Immune System

I went with nineteen members of the "alternative" medicine community to the White House on March 18, 1993, to give formal advice to the White House Task Force on Health Care Reform. For the first time since 1909 — since the Flexner Report ended the growth of homeopathy and installed allopathy as the dominant form of medicine in the United States — alternative medicine had a respectful hearing at the highest levels of our government.

ROBERT M. DUGGAN, *president of the Traditional Acupuncture Institute*

Questions about alternative therapies in relation to the immune system first arose for me as I got to know one of my HIV+ buddies, Bernard. Bernard was a twenty-five-year-old white man from a working-class family who, to make ends meet, had worked as a prostitute from time to time in a nearby city. He was touchingly gentle and sweet and terrified about what was happening to him. Two other women volunteers, attracted by his charm and his need, and I, as his official buddy, became his steady companions. We brought him homemade soup, gave him massages, got him whatever junk food he craved, and kept fresh flowers on his bedside table. His family seldom visited and failed to clear an outstanding phone bill so that he could, as he desperately desired, have a phone hooked up by his bed in the nursing home.

Not long after I began to visit him regularly, he asked me if I could arrange for him to see an acupuncturist. He had read an article about acupuncture and treatment of HIV in the local paper and thought that he would like to give it a try. He said that he wanted it to "fix my head." He explained that his head did not hurt exactly but that he wanted it to feel better, in some way he found hard to put into words. A call to a center for acupuncture treatment near Baltimore eventually led me to Patricia O'Hara, a local acupuncturist who had treated other HIV patients. Patricia set up a schedule to visit Bernard in the nursing home and treat him there.

Patricia understood treatment as enabling Bernard to be at peace as his death approached. She took his request to "fix my head" to mean that he wanted to bring his mental attitudes and feelings into harmony with the inexorable process of dying taking place in his body. Bernard professed to like his treatments and always said that they made his head feel better. About two months later, when I called Patricia to tell her that Bernard had died peacefully during the night while two of his buddies held him, she reflected on the effect of her treatment. Her goal in treating Bernard had been to facilitate the process of his dying, allowing it to come with less anguish: "He was so young and basically healthy before HIV that he could have lasted a long, long time. When I first saw him, he was holding on so tight. He could have suffered a lot longer." In this case, death was taken not as a failure but, since it happened relatively rapidly and peacefully, as a success.

This glimpse into alternative therapies indicated to me that their goals run deeply counter to those of biomedicine. Certainly, Bernard's family never stopped insisting that he be given the latest experimental scientific medicines so that he would be cured—although they did so from afar. Certainly, the nursing home took it as given that Bernard's various maladies should be cured by biomedical means, his eye infection and bed sores treated — even though, because of financial constraints, measures to achieve these cures seldom took place. Only Patricia's goal, unacceptable to either family or doctors, allowed her treatment to focus on something other than a "cure." I decided to gather more material on the views and practices of alternative therapists to see if my initial impressions about their distance from biomedicine would be borne out.

In this chapter, I explore the views of health practitioners who define themselves as in some way "alternative" to standard Western biomedicine. The practitioners we met, observed, and interviewed were not chosen to constitute a representative sample in the scientific sense.[1] But they did give us twelve different views of biomedicine from one point or another outside the mainstream, and they are all active practitioners in the urban area where we conducted fieldwork. We met them through people we interviewed in neighborhoods, by attending local conferences and conventions on alternative health, and by visiting local clinics specifically for alternative practitioners.

Given Patricia's very different approach to Bernard's death, I was surprised to find that "alternative" practitioners' views of health and the body are — as they see them — fundamentally congruent with views emerging in some, but not all, parts of biomedicine. This remarkable confluence in what might otherwise be presumed to be two competing points of view is brought about by way of the immune system.[2]

The immune system serves as an entirely compatible link, a seamless weld, really, between biomedicine and alternative therapies.[3] The alternative practitioners we interviewed often began by stating the incompatibility between what they are doing and what biomedicine is trying to do: many described the "split" that occurred in biomedicine between the mind and the body. Identifying microbes as the cause of certain diseases led to an emphasis on finding miracle cures. As for alternative therapies, they are based on a "completely different viewpoint": a "holistic point of view"; "the whole idea of the mind and the body having some sort of relationship and connection" (Allan Browner, homeopathic M.D.).

In the next breath, many therapists went on to encompass the immune system within whatever alternative method they were using. For example, a nutritionist told us that every cell in the body is an immune system cell. For him, it then follows that massaging the skin will affect the immune system: "Touch. The therapeutic touch, far more healing than anything else. And the part about the immune system is if every cell is an immune cell, then the largest surface area of cells is the skin. Then following that logic, if you give yourself a sesame oil massage, you are activating more immune cells or potential immune cells than any other part of your body" (Frank Saviano).

Moving in the reverse direction, a "holistic physician," an M.D., interpreted his treatments to desensitize his patients' immune systems to things causing an allergic reaction as a form of homeopathy. In homeopathic terms, he treats the illness with a very dilute form of something that is known to cause the illness. In immunological terms, he is desensitizing the immune system:

> Well, I look upon the immunotherapy as a form of homeopathy. . . . It's basically finding the dilution that tells the immune system not to react.
> *OK. Now, is the level of dilution similar to the one in home-opathy? Because the dilution levels are extremely high.*
> Well, when we start, let's say we diagnose a child as being allergic to corn. We will start with each dilution being five times weaker. . . . So we usually start with a number two. See, if reaction develops on the skin or test, depending on the individual, under the tongue or sublingually, so if we get a reaction on the skin — positive reaction — or provoke something in behavior, then we go to the next dilution. So it's basically the principles of homeopathy. You're trying to find the proper dilution that the immune system will accept. (Hugh Millner)

Acupuncturists in particular found it easy to encompass the immune system as a subsidiary component within a set of interlocked systems:

> I think the immune system is contained as a concept within what from an acupuncture perspective would be a person's general energy level or a person's general energy quality. So what I mean to say is that when a person's life force, when a person's "ch'i" energy is flowing smoothly and harmoniously through the person, they are balanced, and balance in the system is equal to relative health. When a person's "ch'i" is flowing smoothly and harmoniously, they'll be exposed to certain bacteria, [but . . .] they're not going to get sick, and their system is going to be able to ward off the bacteria and be strong enough within itself to have the bacteria not affect them in such a way. (Anthony Humphreys)

> *OK. Now, how does your understanding of the immune system fit into this concept of body and health as it is in acupuncture?*
> Somehow, it doesn't feel contradictory. I think I can blend them. You wear gloves, but then you also get acupuncture treat-

ment so your immune system is beefed up, and you're not
going to catch as much of what's coming along as you might.
(Patricia O'Hara)

Alternative therapists can easily enfold the immune system within
various larger wholes. In so doing they are not necessarily subordinat-
ing the immune system to other systems but simply asserting that the
immune system taken alone or in isolation gives far from the whole
picture:

> What's happening with the psychoneuroimmunology movement
> is a recognition that that system does not live isolated — that in
> fact it is integrated into larger wholes, among which are the neu-
> ropeptide system, the autonomic and central nervous system, the
> brain, the hypothalamus, the interpretive — the cortex, which
> deals with emotions and feelings and perceptions and stress.[4] And
> so there is a movement up to a more holistic view of what immu-
> nity is about. . . . That is, if you make a change in stress, or this or
> that, what is the result on the immune system? . . . But there are
> other levels that [psychoneuroimmunology] hasn't really pushed
> through. It hasn't looked more strongly at social support (there
> has been some work in that). It hasn't looked at the effect of
> economy, the work site. It hasn't looked at the issues of nonlocal
> healing. That's the ability of prayer or other such things to heal at
> distances which would not make the physical effect the dominant
> effect. It has not looked at the role of spirituality. (Peter Boswell)

> I'm wondering whether the approach in conventional medicine
> isn't trying to create something out of its individual parts which
> it can never do. Because there's more to a tomato, as an example,
> than just the individual parts. There's a whole integrated func-
> tion. And I think the immune system is like that. It's the expres-
> sion of the [whole] that holds a life form together. (Thomas
> Womack)

These statements clearly show us how easily the nesting of the immune
system in larger wholes can be done, but the details of that nesting can
vary. A student of acupuncture conceives it like this: "We don't live as
separate islands, we live in a bigger system called 'the globe,' and people will expand that to the universe, as well. In order to really be

healthy, you need to be at one with the seasons. . . . This concept of interrelationships is integral to this system, the philosophical sense of the Tao, the philosophical sense that everything is connected. So, in that sense, it is our own energy, and yet our own energy is more one expression of a bigger energy" (Anthony Humphreys).

For Martin Rabinow, an M.D. who practices nutritional medicine, the immune system is "only one portion of the whole picture." He is not sure where one would draw boundaries around the immune system and say that another part of the person lies outside it. Even the skeletal system might be considered part of the immune system because it protects us from collapsing. Perhaps, he wonders, medicine tries to set the immune system off from the rest of the whole only because it is quantifiable, it has features that we can measure.

Throughout these therapists' accounts, the immune system, and every system in which it is embedded, is consistently represented as being in a constant process of change:

> And he [Deepok Chopra in *Quantum Healing* (1989)] says that
> his explanation of what I'm gonna tell you parallels why the
> alternative healing works, why homeopathy and Bach flowers
> and massage and art healing and any one you can think of,
> acupuncture, all of them work. Number one, he says, this
> [pointing to his body] is our universe. It's the same as the uni-
> verse out there.
> **OK.**
> OK. So it ebbs and flows like the tides of [the ocean]. The sun
> rises, it sets. Things change. That's how our body works. Now to
> try and change that is like trying to make it stop
> raining. (Frank Saviano)

> My personal concept of health is not anything static. . . . To be
> statically healthy is impossible because there is, sort of, no such
> thing as static, because every second we're changing, every sec-
> ond I take a different breath, every second the air quality in the
> room changes, so it's an interplay between health and not-
> health. And, as I see it, the great goal for a person, in terms of
> their health, is not to be statically healthy, just to have the ups
> and downs be closer to center. So the image that I have is of a
> seesaw. (Anthony Humphreys)

When we asked these practitioners to reflect on the common use of military metaphors to describe the immune system, they were very quick to suggest other ways of thinking about the matter. An M.D. practicing homeopathic medicine explained that health is a matter not of obliterating pathogens but of establishing a balance with them, of keeping them in the right place and proportion: "I think that every person is exposed to a wide variety of different pathogens. That if you just look at bowel flora, if any of them gets out of hand — out of balance — it can easily result in disease. Even quite normal flora in an abnormal place. So the body is constantly striving to maintain balance, to keep those areas of the body that need to be separated, from each other, not only separated, but functioning and interacting in a balanced fashion" (Thomas Womack).

Discussing the cover of *Time* magazine, an acupuncturist suggests as an alternative the metaphor of health as the body's rivers flowing without interruption: "Acupuncture would look at this and think 'Ah, this person has some kind of aggressive energy, we have to drain it.'. . . My metaphor would be rivers that are flowing without interruption, without being dammed up. When we get an illness, it's a bit of a dammed up area, and so to allow that area to flow again, we dose it with antibiotics or some type of energy intervention. So I guess that's the metaphor I'd like to use" (Patricia O'Hara). In place of fights and battles or opposition between self and nonself, a student of acupuncture suggests building bridges and establishing a healthy meeting place: "Building a bridge between the outside and the inside, as opposed to keeping anything out, so to speak. It's more about a healthy meeting of the two, is the best way to say it. I think it's more about a healthy meeting of the outside and the inside as opposed to keeping it out because, of course, it's going to be coming in" (Anthony Humphreys).

An M.D. with an interest in psychoneuroimmunology accepts the centrality of defense and fighting in the activities of the immune system but insists that this activity simultaneously links us to all other organisms: the immune system simultaneously sets us off from the nonself and links us to it:

> I suppose what the immune system fundamentally does is distinguish self from nonself. . . . To the extent that its design has a universality about it, it is also a mark of interconnectedness. . . . The immune system is basically a violent, aggressive, and hostile system — it's not a very friendly one, in a sense. And so it tells me

that in our biology, perhaps in our psyche, instinctually, we do carry a deep sense of self and nonself, of survival, destructiveness, of aggressiveness and hostility, as well as a transcendent quality, connectedness and spirituality, in that it is an undeniable statement about the duality — duality and polarity of life. (Peter Boswell)

What is striking about these interviews is that *all* the alternative practitioners in one way or another asserted the inadequacy of models that see the body as a defended fortress set apart from and at war with the rest of the world. All of them also elaborated a vision of health as a condition in which the great number of elements in a complex system are being sufficiently well managed in relation to each other.

A study recently published in the *New England Journal of Medicine* showed the extent to which Americans use alternative therapies: one of three respondents did so in the past year. Extrapolating to the U.S. population it was estimated that "in 1990 Americans made an estimated 425 million visits to providers of unconventional therapy. This number exceeds the number of visits to all U.S. primary care physicians (388 million). Expenditures associated with use of unconventional therapy in 1990 amounted to approximately $13.7 billion, three quarters of which ($10.3 billion) was paid out of pocket. This figure is comparable to the $12.8 billion spent out of pocket annually for all hospitalizations in the United States" (Eisenberg et al.1993:246). The editorial accompanying this article adopts a scolding tone toward patients who spend so much money on such therapies, many of which are based on theories that are "quackery" or "patently unscientific," and do not tell their doctors (Campion 1993).

It would be a mistake to read these figures as a response to the health care crisis addressed by the Clinton administration because the study was conducted before the crisis had become a national issue. Of course, one issue that led to the crisis — cost containment — may have played a role in determining the kind of health care people seek: not insignificantly, alternative practitioners' services are often less expensive than those of biomedical practitioners. But, in addition to lower cost, another factor should be considered.

What is really at issue in the increasing numbers of people visiting alternative practitioners is not medical fraud or charlatanry but the incompatibility between biomedicine's view of the body and the immune system and the views of many nonmedical people. Alternative practices offer a place where the complex systems thinking that so commonly accompanies how people talk about the immune system can meet with an enthusiastic response, a response that is able to subordinate biomedicine by incorporating it.[5]

In 1977, George Engel, a professor of psychiatry and medicine, set out the main characteristics of biomedicine in the following terms: "The biomedical model embraces both reductionism, the philosophic view that complex phenomena are ultimately derived from a single primary principle, and mind-body dualism, the doctrine that separates the mental from the somatic. Here the reductionistic primary principle is physicalistic; that is, it assumes that the language of chemistry and physics will ultimately suffice to explain biological phenomena" (Engel 1977:130). Engel thought that this model was the "dominant folk model of disease in the Western world," and, looking back from the time he wrote toward the past, he was probably right. He also anticipated the importance of systems thinking for developing a different view of health and disease, arguing that a systems approach would enable physicians and medical scientists to encompass a biopsychosocial perspective on disease. He could not have anticipated that the *non*-scientists we met in Chapter 2 and the alternative practitioners we met in this chapter would have arrived at a point far ahead on Engel's trajectory before, as we will see in the next chapter, much of biomedicine did.

CHAPTER 4

Immunophilosophy: How Scientists See the Immune System

In comparative epistemology, cognition must not be construed as only a dual relationship between the knowing subject and the object to be known. The existing fund of knowledge must be a third partner in this relation as a basic factor of all new knowledge.
    LUDWIK FLECK, *Genesis and Development of a Scientific Fact*

One of the clearest moments of "implosion" in my fieldwork, when elements from different research contexts seemed to collapse into one another with great force, occurred in a graduate course I was taking on immunology.[1] Having guided us through many weeks of introductory material, the professor finally began to talk in detail about the heart of the immune system, the cells that produce a specific immune response against something foreign in the body. When a B cell gets the proper signal, he said, it starts to produce quantities of highly specific antibodies designed to lock with great precision to the foreign material. The kinds of antibodies that are produced in advance is staggeringly large in number, a feat achieved through

91

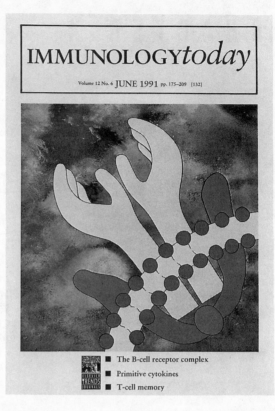

IMMUNOLOGY*today*

Volume 12 No. 6 JUNE 1991 pp. 175–209 [132]

■ The B-cell receptor complex
■ Primitive cytokines
■ T-cell memory

Fig. 19. *The antibody shown as hands on a B cell on the cover of* Immunology Today. *From* Immunology Today, *vol. 12, no. 6 (June 1991). Reprinted with permission of the publisher.*

genetic mutation; those selected to counter a particular kind of foreign matter he described as "exquisitely specific" or "tailor-made." But — and here is where the implosion occurred for me — accompanying this exquisite specificity is also the ability to be "flexible." The professor held up his hand to illustrate: the two ends of the Y-shaped antibody are specific to the "keys" on the foreign material that it must match, but the antibody can bend and adjust at the hinge region as it moves in. It is therefore flexible *and* specific. The professor flexed his wrist and moved his thumb back and forth to meet his fingers to illustrate the possibilities.[2] A cover of the professional journal *Immunology Today* graphically pictures the flexibly specific "hands" of an antibody (see fig. 19).

I learned later that the discovery of the flexibility of the antibody was a galvanizing moment in the development of immunology. Nobel Prize–winner Gerald Edelman recalls the "shock of molecular recognition" that he experienced when he first saw an electron micrograph of an antibody, which revealed its floppy Y shape, its flexibility. He recalls that he should have listened earlier to colleague Al Nisonoff, who told him that the molecule could not have the "cigar" shape that Edelman favored because, "after all, it must attach to things and have room to interact" (Edelman 1975:9, 17).[3]

In my mind, this language crashed into contemporary descriptions of the economy of the late twentieth century (mentioned in Part II), with a focus on flexible specialization, flexible production, and flexible, rapid response to an ever-changing market with specific, tailor-made products. Was I watching as the images developing in scientists' minds incorporated, *within* the body, models of a system and how its parts interact that is being given great salience by forces in the society at large? Or was I watching as scientists gave life to a biological model that went out *from* science into the society and in turn enlivened our general concepts of what it takes to make a robust organization? Or were these models arising completely independently of each other? The course on immunology made me want to know much more about how scientists see their work fitting into daily life and how they imagine the world inside the body.

THE LAB AND DAILY LIFE

My participant-observation took place mainly in one research group in a department of immunology with about a dozen such research subgroups. In order to include the perspectives of scientists outside my group and department, we interviewed over forty scientists in other departments who used immunological knowledge in their research, teaching, or clinical practice. Perhaps because these scientists were all biologists and most were closely involved with clinical problems, if not actual clinics and patients, the ambience of these places of work was very different from the isolated atmosphere that other observers have described in physical science laboratories. According to Karin Knorr-Cetina (personal communication), for example, a physicist in the lab where she did fieldwork might work alongside other physicists for years on the same research apparatus and never even know whether his colleagues were married.[4]

Observers have commented on scientists in the physical sciences having an obsessive and exclusionary involvement with their machines out of a need to exert a kind of masculine control over them (Turkle 1984; Traweek 1988:158–59). Not only did I not feel any similar climate, but it is hard to imagine how one could develop. Immunologists have to orchestrate a wide variety of instruments, organic substances, reagents, animals, people, and their body fluids, scientific models, administrators, and funding agencies to carry on their work.[5] Issues involving work in the lab covered the whole gamut: could sufficient samples of HIV+ human blood be obtained from the clinic? Were the frozen samples of mouse blood with certain antibodies in danger of degradation? Would a new graduate student arrive in time to carry out an essential part of an experiment before a grant application had to be complete?

For that matter, one of the key experimental techniques used in the lab in which I worked, the Western blot, was often the cause of lament rather than obsessive delight because of its sheer, unavoidable blurriness. Are the bands that would show the presence of an antibody *there*? Are we seeing them or imagining them? Can we convince our colleagues that they *are* there? One of my mentors commented, "Western blots do not look exactly great in a photograph [for a publication]."

In the immunology department of my research, daily life outside the lab was a frequent companion. I quickly learned the basic life circumstances of most of the people with whom I worked, from career plans to wedding plans, just by participating in and overhearing casual conversation. I do not think that I was treated in an atypically relaxed and informal way because of my status as an anthropologist. If anything, my presence occasionally seemed to make people feel on their guard, as when the person about to present a paper at a seminar saw me and said, "Oh, no, this will be recorded for posterity." Nor could the informality that I observed be put down to prior friendships between me and lab members: I had never met anyone in the lab or the larger department before my research.

The immediate small research group, about even numbers of men and women, often ate lunch together in the department seminar room or a nearby market and discussed problems ranging from carrying out an experiment in the lab to buying a house or redecorating a room at home. Major life events like weddings would certainly lead to a lab party, but so might smaller events such as birthdays. Children of lab members would occasionally appear on days when they had no school and wander curiously about the offices and hallways. The technicians told me, "Things here are very friendly, like a family really." Discussions about the immune system itself also did not seem to me unduly narrow. One of my main mentors, Peter VanHorn, seemed to enjoy our broad-ranging discussions about the way he saw the immune system operating and began to refer to them as *immunophilosophy*.[6]

This porousness with respect to the world outside the lab does not appear to be atypical of immunology. In 1986, a group of immunologists devoted an entire conference to discussions of "immunosemiotics" (Sercarz et al. 1988). There were a number of semioticians at the conference, including Umberto Eco (author of the novel *The Name of the Rose*); one of them gave the flavor of how fruitful the linkage between the two fields was:

> The reason for discussing semiotics at this meeting of immunologists is the fact of being faced with a strange situation: Immunologists are forced to use unusual expressions in order to describe their observations. Expressions like "memory," "recognition," "interpretation," "individuality," "reading," "inner picture," "self," "nonself," . . . or "killing"— to list only some of them — are unknown in physics and chemistry. Atoms and molecules have no self, memory, individuality, or inner pictures. They are not able to read, to recognise or to interpret anything and cannot be killed either. This means that it is not possible to solve the problems described with these expressions by translating them into physical or chemical processes or explaining them in physical or chemical terms. (Uexküll 1988:25)

More personal connections between immunological research and daily life outside were less clear. Only a few (five) of the approximately forty scientists we interviewed said that they often made connections between the research they carried out in the lab and their own health. These few mentioned attending to their diet, amount of sleep or exercise, or vaccinations. Only one person said that he actually thought about the immune system, antibodies, T cells, etc. when he was fighting off a cold or suffering from the flu. Sometimes scientists said that they avoided trying to apply their scientific knowledge because they knew too much: "My view is that I'm aware of many of those things but it could ruin my life if I always just fixated on it" (Vivian Becker).

Out of too much knowledge can come fear, denial, and inaction:

> As for my health, I'm an absolute denier. I don't see doctors. I avoid them like the plague, except as fellow professionals, and I

rarely, if ever, see to my own health so that, you know, a couple of years ago, I had a retinal detachment, which is within my purview. I mean, I know about retinal detachments and basically apparently ignored it for six to eight months before just casually asking somebody to take a look at it. . . . I know what can go wrong, and I'd rather just not address it. You know, if I die, I die. (Ron Wilder)

The ease with which nonscientists and alternative practitioners connect the immune system to other things, indeed, to *everything* else, contrasts starkly to these scientists' reluctance to see connections between the object of their research and their own daily lives. In part this may be due to their acceptance of a common, idealized picture of science as abstract, separate, and above the concrete, mundane world of everyday events.

INSIDE THE IMMUNE SYSTEM

As for the object of their research itself, the immune system, most scientists we interviewed described it in terms of the body at war, which established a common ground between them and the popular media as well as some nonscientists.[7] Many people asserted that this image is not just a metaphor but "how it is." Even Guy Lerchen, who personally was not attracted by military imagery, felt that there was no better way to describe the immune system:

It's a pretty harsh world, that immune system. . . . I mean, these lymphocytes see something they don't like, and they arrive at the scene, and they inject nasty chemicals onto it. They attack it, leave it obliterated, have their mop-up crew come by and chew it all up. It's pretty harsh.
How else could you think of it? How about a guess?
I mean, it's not like, "Let's come to a consensus," like, you know, the virus comes in, and lymphocytes hang out and, say, talk to the lawyers and say, "Let's be reasonable about this, you know. I think you should go back home." . . . No reasonable discussions take place in the immune system. . . . The reason I don't like the military metaphor is because I think we're fighting wrong battles, militarily.
Yeah? For example?

Our involvement in Iraq. But this, I think, is a pretty legitimate war. I mean, if you knew a virus was going to come in and kill you, I think it's self-defense.
So it's —
A just war.

But there are many other ways in which these scientists modified and blunted the ability of the military metaphor to describe the immune system. Ron Wilder regards military images as very simplistic because they relate only to times when the immune system becomes intensely mobilized: "When I talk to my patients, I tell them, I'm giving you a very simple, abbreviated, cartoon version. The immune system has nonwarfare roles in maintaining your body. I mean, it does things even when you're not fighting a war and there's not a battle inside your body. But the metaphor is easy to communicate. It gets people's attention, and people tend to remember it long after they cease to remember all the precise data. So I agree with it as long as you're honest about the fact that this is very simplistic." He also negates the choice of a military war as the only appropriate image by pouring out a whole list of other images at the drop of a hat:

> *OK. Now would you think of another metaphor that could be used and maybe would be not as reductionist?*
> Yeah. You could use such metaphors as the symphony metaphor: that in a symphony you have woodwinds and you have percussionists and all that. These are not [in] conflict, but each of them are doing their own little specialized jobs to achieve a goal and that at one level there's some T cells (that's the conductor), the B cells are the percussions, etc. You can use that kind of a metaphor. You could use the corporate metaphor: that the body is divided into a bunch of divisions and each division has a production quota and that kind of thing. You can use economic metaphors. So there's lots of metaphors that can be used. I suppose even the nurturing mother metaphor, [where] the immune system is like your mom that only makes sure that you get good food, eliminates all the bad food, and that sort of thing.
> *OK. So there're plenty of ideas. Now why do you think the military metaphor is still the prevailing one? You said it's because people understand conflict.*

That's partly it. The other part of it though is that most people
tend to think of their immune systems mainly in connection
with disease. That if you're fine, you don't care about your
immune system, really. That the only time people tend to really
think of their immune system is when they have the flu, when
they have cancer, when they have AIDS or somebody they
know has AIDS. So by that time we're already dealing with a
very deranged time in the life of the immune system. Most of
the time the immune system's in balance, but in these cases, the
immune system is off to the edge doing something. It's sort of
like saying you look at history, history tends to concentrate on
wars and treaties. Ninety-nine percent of the time, Belgians
weren't fighting wars, and they weren't writing treaties. They're
just doin' their thing: selling, eating, whatever. But if you read
your history books, you read about — we had this war, we
signed that treaty. Because those are sort of highlights that people think about and remember. But most of the time Americans
and Belgians weren't doing anything of that much moment. It's
the same way with the immune system. The military metaphor
is an attractive one because it captures the moment when people are most interested in their immune systems.

In other words, the military account of the immune system pre-
serves and gives emphasis to certain sorts of events: the equivalent of
a traditional history of generals, battles, and their dates. Most of the
time, the immune system (as well as any society in the history books)
goes about carrying on daily life, the mundane business of feeding and
clothing and cleaning its members —"doin' its thing." Ken Holden
makes almost the same point in different words:

It's like history. Until the recent past, when they were doing
archaeological findings into armies and fortresses and citadels
and everything, that's the first thing you see. You see invasions,
you see massacres, you see pillages. Now, if you start looking a
little more deeply, you realize that, behind the wars, there is a
society. And, in the immune system, it's the same thing. You see
diseases; these are the wars. You see the tools, the antibodies.
And you see the reactions against antibodies and all that. So that's
the first level. Now we're actually starting to understand what's
below. And below there are a million other things, and there are

all sorts of cells that are actually never taking part in the fight. So, what are these? You know, when Napoléon goes all the way to Moscow and makes his battles, I mean, there is a whole society behind that feeds him. I mean, these guys are also important because if he doesn't have millions of peasants to feed his army, where does he go? So the immune system is the same thing. So the military metaphor is interesting. It's good, it was probably excellent at some point, it's maybe not so excellent at this point.

It is as if the contemporary movement to rewrite traditional history to include cultural and social factors ("history from below") is circling back here to affect the metaphors found appropriate to describe the immune system. But, if one way to make the reading of the military metaphor more complex is to regard it as only a partial account of the body's activities, another way, as we saw in the last chapter, is to change the description of the metaphoric war that the immune system is to fight. Ken Holden continues:

> We used to look at it in terms of traditional war, as opposed to how people talk about the Gulf War, where a very minute amount of the people were actually involved in fighting, and probably none of them saw the enemy in the eyes. Almost all the effort, all the money went into technology, communication, satellite trans- mission of data, gathering of information. And that was what made the war. OK? As opposed to the Iraqi army. . . . Now, some- body [who] doesn't know about computers and doesn't know satellites would look at the Allied army in the Gulf and see it as being pretty similar to the Iraqi army. Now, if you know that com- puters exist, then you look inside the tank, you find a computer; inside the plane, you find another computer. If you look in space, you find a satellite. And then behind all that, there is an entire society that's got to produce all these things. So it's an evolving view.

Another approach to describing the immune system is to reject mil- itary imagery altogether, as Robert Davies did. Stating, "I'm very paci- fistic, I wouldn't have a military," he proceeded to develop an account of the immune system that was phrased entirely in terms of a commu- nication system: elements in the system "orchestrate," "recognize," "present," "activate," "turn on or off."

Another way to dislodge the military metaphor is to question the basis for the choice of that image in the first place. The basis for choosing military metaphors is said to be that they maintain a sharp, clear boundary between self, which is to be kept in, and nonself, which is to be kept out. In my role as a student of immunology, I was told in a variety of ways that maintaining the integrity of the system (distinguishing self from nonself) is the most fundamental concept in modern immunology.

But many of the scientists we interviewed, even those who were enthusiastic about the military metaphor, could see its limitations. Guy Lerchen, who described the immune system as a "just war," added afterward that the immune system "allows a certain level of foreign things" in a kind of symbiosis. Other scientists took the notion of symbiosis much farther:

> There's this mechanistic notion about how the body works, and frequently the body is considered actually to be a machine. And the machine metaphor always has the implication that parts of the machine can go awry and that those parts can be replaced and it's only a crummy mechanic who can't find the carburetor or who can't get this bolt undone. In the hands of a confident mechanic there should be total health. Very little is given to the idea that it's actually a very dynamic system that has a million levels of control and is not readily understood in mechanistic terms. . . . But it's entirely possible that the viruses and the immune system and us have all co-evolved to allow viruses to do important things — for example, rearrange the genome or something like that. So viruses . . . would jump into genes or jump out of genes and cause mutations or somehow affect the organization of the genome. And so, yes, the immune system in the military metaphor fights the viruses, but maybe actually they don't fight in a regular military sense, but somehow it's more like mutual or shared destruction or something like that where there's a détente of sorts where the immune system actually lets the virus do some things but doesn't let it do other things. (Bruce Kleiner)

As he begins to think about it, Allan Chase works through some of the limitations of the military analogy and thinks of an alternative, even though he has never seen it used:

You can't actually talk about — you're right! You cannot talk about the immune system in English without using what are military analogies.
Can you think of a different analogy?
Yeah, I mean, I can, but it's not one I've ever seen. I could think of saying that your body's immune system functions as an interface between the human body and the environment. . . . I mean, that's a way of saying that you automatically are going to interact with your environment, and there are certain things that are hostile to the human body, and you can understand how the metaphor was generated, the "defense" and everything. But actually, if you think about it, it gets a little carried away. . . . "The immune system wages a battle. . . . " You should find textbooks; I'm sure there's probably a hundred examples that you could pluck out of textbooks . . . and there's a lot of really violent immunologic imagery that's used. It's interesting . . . you wonder if it's not, in a way, to rev people up, y'know. "My body's hard at work doing battle against the external environment." (Allan Chase)

When it comes to the cells that make up the immune system and the special character of each, those scientists who were attached to the view that the immune system is basically a military defense system that protects the integrity of our body boundaries were likely to describe the cells in a clearly hierarchical ranking. For example, Mitchell Woodruff arranged the cells with the T cell at the top, the B cell next, and the macrophage, the most primitive, at the bottom. In many ways, other people conveyed this same ranking. Reminiscent of the media views, these scientists admire T cells for their ability to move, to have free rein of the body (Bruce Kleiner). A T cell is likened to a fullback (Richard Walton), the conductor of the immune orchestra (Michael O'Grady), the "main specific protagonist who regulates all" (Mitchell Woodruff). The "real guts [of the immune system], the general, [who] determines self, [and is] capable of killing cells in its own right" (Martin Greiber).

The macrophages are made to seem inferior in many ways: they are like garbage collectors (Guy Lerchen), they cannot distinguish self from nonself and so are not critical to the immune system (Claude Tanner), they are nonspecific (Michael O'Grady), they are "big, amorphous, protoplasmic blobs" (Martin Greiber). Perhaps most important,

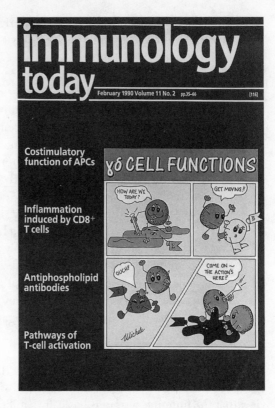

Fig. 20. *T cells and B cells as dominant males and subordinate females on the cover of* Immunology Today. *From* Immunology Today, *vol. 11, no. 2 (February 1990). Reprinted with permission of the publisher.*

macrophages do not have the capacity to "name," "identify," "categorize," the nature of the things they indiscriminately gobble up. Like a young child who will pick anything up from the gutter, they lack the highly valued ability to identify the bits of matter they encounter. Ron Wilder makes it very clear: macrophages "take off small pieces of what they eat and put those pieces on their cell membranes along with other molecules to attract the notice of T cells (to some extent B cells) and say, 'Hey, I've got something that's gross here. Eliminate it, please.'" In Robert Davies's words, "They're kind of not very smart, and they're nonspecific, and they go around, and they eat everything in sight." In these accounts, as in the media examples discussed in Chapter 1, macrophages are given all the characteristics of "lower-class" stereotypes: they are slovenly, immature, unsophisticated, and out of shape.

The cartoon on a recent cover of the technical journal *Immunology Today* provides clear evidence for the picture that I am drawing (see fig. 20). This cartoon depicts a B cell drawn with long eyelashes and high heels, silently taking orders from a T cell called a gamma/delta cell, drawn as a doctor with a stethoscope and a hypodermic needle. As the "male" gamma/delta T cell gives his order —"Get moving!!"— he kicks the "female" B cell with a smile. In the next frame, the gamma/delta T cell (now frowning manfully) kicks another kind of T cell unmarked by any adornments, but this T cell registers a verbal protest —"Ouch!!" In the final frame, two gamma/delta T cells are shown standing on top of a macrophage, while one of them shouts into a megaphone, "Come on — the action's here!!" (Born et al. 1990).

Although some scientists were enthusiastic about developing a military hierarchy, others evinced the most fervent interest in the ability of the immune system to produce a large number of highly specific antibodies that lock perfectly into foreign proteins and thus signal further response from the immune system. Again and again in our interviews, these laboratory scientists echoed the excitement of my professor about the wondrous capacities of the flexible but specific antibody, the "tailor-made" antibody:[8]

> The B cell's basic job is to synthesize a protein molecule called *immunoglobulin*, also known as *antibodies*. All right. Basically, what an antibody does is it interacts with a foreign protein in the same way that a key interacts with a lock, or the same way a baseball glove fits around a baseball, or whatever you want to say. And, basically, a foreign organism like a bacterium, or a virus, or whatever, its going to have its own proteins on its surface, its own unique proteins. . . . What a B cell's gonna do is under the direction of a T cell. The B cell is going to manufacture an antibody which is going to fit specifically onto one of the proteins on the invading organism. Now how does that help us? Well, antibodies do two things. Antibodies actually have two combining sites in them, sort of like a pitchfork or something with two prongs on them. And basically, since it can combine with two things, it can actually hook two cells together, and the other end can like hook more cells together, and what you can basically do is you can agglutinate the invader and get him all balled up and gummed up into one big bulb so they can't go out, and it makes it more easily destroyed. (Martin Greiber)

Dan Marshak got so exhilarated that he acted out the role of the antibody, using his own arms and legs:

So they float around. Picture me with my arms floating around, with my two arms. I see something I don't recognize. I see something which my hands are being made to bind to, grab onto it. I grab onto it, and I start wiggling my leg. And that's the message, and so I'm like wiggling my leg. [Laughs.] And there's a bunch of us like me bobbing on this thing, wiggling our legs, and this big IGM molecule [another type of antibody] sees all these wiggling legs and binds onto that.

Robert Davies calls the matching process "pretty miraculous," and Guy Lerchen develops the image of "sticky hands" to describe the very precise matching between antibody and antigen, followed by an "incredible" response:

I have this picture of . . . these surveillance cells that are just swimming everywhere, looking for foreign objects. And then, you know, they just, kind of, are actually going around feeling, just kind of feeling out their environment constantly, day in and day out, twenty-four hours a day. And then, sometimes, you know, they have, like, sticky hands . . . but very specific sticky hands. Like, antibodies are so specific that you have one specific antibody for each possible foreign object. So, once its hand actually grabs something that's specifically like a lock in the key, you know, it just sets off this incredible response, where this cell, which is secreting this antibody to kill this one thing, starts multiplying out of control.
Wow.

Some scientists, building on the notion that immune system cells "feel" each other out with their "very specific sticky hands," demolished the whole idea of a hierarchy among them. For example, Martin Greiber asserted that the role of each cell was equally important and that their interaction was a collaboration. Sarah Gaspari said that the T cell can "feel" the difference between self and nonself. It has "nice little hands" on it and knows what self feels like. But the T cell needs to be able to "feel" something foreign, and, until it "feels" it on the surface of an appropriate cell, the T cell will not know it is foreign. T cells usually "feel" the bits of foreign things when they are presented on the surfaces of macrophages and B cells, cells that have been able to *see* foreign things. This amounts to saying that the T cell has a developed sense of touch but cannot *see*, suggesting that it is dependent on other cells, macrophages and B cells, for its "vision." A picture of mutual dependence among the cells of the immune system emerges here.

One scientist muses on the shift in perspective that now allows greater appreciation of the importance of the macrophage, even though "the leaders in the field of immunology are not working on macrophages. . . . The people who are mostly considered to be the giants in the field work on problems related to B cells and T cells." Even though macrophages cannot distinguish self from nonself as T cells can, he continues,

> Macrophages do produce a large number of what are called *cytokines* that affect the behavior of other cells. And this is the major part of their activity and of their role that I would say ten years ago was probably not much appreciated, because very few cytokines were identified. But now that many cytokines are identified, it turns out that the macrophage is really quite an amazing cell in its ability to produce a large number of these things. And these molecules not only have importance for the function of the immune system, and are practically important in that sense, but because they are secreted molecules, they have potential medical importance because they are molecules that can be used as drugs or that can be inhibited by giving drugs. . . . And the macrophage is the major source, the sole source of many of these cytokines. What a macrophage does is perhaps not as conceptually challenging as what the T cell does. Nonetheless, it's of great potential practical importance. (Claude Tanner)

Here the shift away from a simple top-down perspective is clear, but the T cells still remain preeminent. Similarly, an immunology graduate student reports: "Well, I haven't thought of it in terms of a hierarchy. I always thought of everything working together. Just subsets sometimes or together. Because macrophages serve a very critical role for the T cells too. So I obviously can't say that I view them as less important. I mean, in terms of functions, direct functions, I think the T cells do have more" (Shelley Borel). Another scientist, however, gives the macrophage its full due:

> The macrophage is a key player in the initiation of a response, and the inability of the macrophage to recognize, encounter,

process, and present the foreign antigen [would] mean that there would be no specific immune response. So that's the key piece. Once that's been accomplished, that sets into motion the things that lead to immunologic memory, thus the response and so forth that allow the individual to be protected from further exposures to the same or even related pathogens.

Now often you will find in textbooks a sort of hierarchy among the immune cells, and then, in general, the T cell is placed at the top and the macrophage at the bottom. I'm sort of interested to know why you don't invert their roles but [instead] seem to be giving to the macrophage a very key and central role.

Well, the macrophage serves as an antigen presenting cell which interacts with both T cells and B cells. And I see that as being probably the most important aspect of the whole interaction. I think perhaps other people place the T cell at the top of the pyramid because T cells can be either effector cells, that is, capable of recognizing and destroying infected cells, or . . . co-participants in eliciting an antibody response. But unless you have the antigen presented in an immunologically meaningful context, then you have no immune response. And so the T cell and B cells are just there waiting to be stimulated, so that's why I would assemble it that way. (Richard Walton)

In one conversation, all the possibilities came together: a blurring of the boundary between self and nonself, a giving up of the hierarchical ranking of immune system cells, and an abandonment of military imagery. This is what emerged in the response of Bruce Kleiner:

Well, I like to think of the body as this standing universe full of all kinds of little creatures, and if you think of it on a cellular level, it's as diverse as the world is in the sense that you have all kinds of citizens in the universe of the body. And some people like to equate the immune system with the police department or the military. That's OK. You can think of that. And just for starters that's not a bad way to think about it. And what they're doing is they're cruising around looking, sniffing for, waiting for distress signals which are usually in the form of some sort of hormone released by cells under attack. But there's probably a better way to think about it or another way to think about it—because with that analogy you get this notion that there are a bunch of idle policemen hanging around on call all the time. And they zip off whenever they can from their little post. But, in fact, it's a little more complicated than that because the immune system is a scavenger system where all the time the integrity between the inside and the outside is violated, like when you have a bowel movement, bacteria get into your blood. I mean, a minute number to be sure, but you can actually measure [it] sometimes. And certainly you can find evidence for it. So you have this wall that separates you from the outside, but it's not 100 percent inviolable. So you find that the immune system is that set of cells whose job it is to scavenge around for trespassers. And they're busy all the time. They're busy. And getting back to the question you talked about — why didn't this person get sick while another did? Well, one other branch of that explanation is that they did get it but they didn't know they got it . . . they were not symptomatic. But the body greeted the stranger and took care of the problem before there was a whole lot of damage done. . . . Probably we're diseased all the time, but we're hardly ever ill. . . . You could think of lymphocytes as buzzards. They're just kind of floating around, and wherever there's a dead rabbit on the side of the road or whatever, they're just going scavenging and recycling and that sort of thing.

By shifting to a new set of defining assumptions, Bruce Kleiner can wonder openly about mysteries in the body. Just as he redefines the roles of all immune cells as scavengers, so he wonders whether there are aspects of T cells that have not been understood: whether their ability to move across blood vessels and "traverse into the depths of the tissues and go into the brain" means "maybe they are whispering in the ears of neurons and then going over to the kidneys exchanging — you never know. There may be other things the immune system's doing that we haven't thought of."

THE FIELD OF IMMUNOLOGY

Bruce Kleiner is a young scientist, relatively near the beginning of his career, which might account for his openness to new descriptions of the immune system. But a very senior immunologist, with whom I had many conversations, was just as willing to explore novel ideas as

well. I often brought him examples of media coverage of the immune
system organized around the image of war. More than once, he commented, disgruntled, "This we owe to microbiology." He meant that
not all biological specialties are alike and that immunologists look at
the world differently. He went on to explain that a freestanding department of immunology is unusual in U.S. universities. More often,
immunology is included along with other "specialties" like virology or
parasitology, under the umbrella of microbiology, rather than being
treated as a separate discipline on a par with microbiology.

I was reminded of biologist Ruth Hubbard's recent statement about
molecular biology: "Most modern biologists believe that work at the
molecular level will yield a more profound understanding of nature
than they could get from the study of cells, organs, or entire organisms.
. . . Molecular biology has therefore become the most prestigious of
the biological disciplines" (Hubbard and Wald 1993:3). It is not that
immunologists do not work at the molecular level, but their conceptu-
alization of the body as a complex system always pulls the part under
scrutiny, even a part at the molecular level, into relation with the whole
system. In classrooms and in conversations, immunologists frequently
expressed their fascination and delight with the ability to discover how
one part of the system affects another, and is in turn affected, until, in
an unimaginably large number of looping, mutual interactions, the
scintillating, ever-changing, adaptive, anticipatory, learning immune
system results.

Just how willing immunologists are to think in terms of complex systems was brought home to me in another conversation with the senior
immunologist, Aaron Hunter. To start off a discussion about the central
distinction between self and nonself, I presented Dr. Hunter with a
section of a paper written by an early immunologist, Ludwik Fleck.
Fleck was a Polish biologist who worked on finding a diagnostic test for
typhus in the 1930s. About immunology, Fleck said:

> The concept of infectious disease is based on the notion of the
> organism as a closed unit and of the hostile causative agents
> invading it. The causative agent produces a bad effect (*attack*).
> The organism responds with a reaction (*defense*). This results in
> a conflict, which is taken to be the essence of disease. The whole
> of immunology is permeated with such primitive images of war.
> . . . But not a single experimental proof exists that could force an
> unbiased observer to adopt such an idea. . . . An organism can no

longer be construed as a self-contained, independent unit with fixed boundaries. . . . In the light of this concept [the harmonious life unit], man appears as a complex to whose harmonious well-being many bacteria, for instance, are absolutely essential. . . . It is very doubtful whether an invasion in the old sense is possible, involving as it does an interference by completely foreign organisms in natural conditions. A completely foreign organism could find no receptors capable of reaction and thus could not generate a biological process. (Fleck [1935] 1979:59–61)

I knew that Dr. Hunter had his doubts about military imagery, but I was astonished to hear him accept Fleck's devastating critique of immunology's current assumptions about the centrality of the self/nonself distinction. He thought that, although most immunologists would take the self/nonself distinction as their starting point, this distinction sometimes gets them into trouble:

If you think just in terms of warfare, it is a little hard to explain autoimmunity, transplantation, why should you battle a leg from someone else, it would do you a lot of good! . . . [Microbes] are not just soldiers attacking us in the sense of attacking the U.S. They are just living their lives because they happen to live their lives in us. Plenty of organisms live their lives happily with us. Warfare is a very nice way to explain it on a very superficial level, but a normal part of existence as microorganisms is balance, so . . . Fleck is right!

What Dr. Hunter's response tells us, significantly, is that the model of the body as sharply bounded along a clear self/nonself line (the model that is so widely described by military, defensive imagery) is actually a model of the body as a simple, mechanical system.

As I explored further in my classes and readings in immunology, I learned that there is a school of thought in contemporary immunology that rejects as inadequate the warfare/defended-self model of the body. This view is inspired by the work of Niels Jerne, published, interestingly enough, at the beginning of the period of flexible specialization. Jerne proposed looking at the immune system as a network of communicating cells that can learn from and adapt to experience. According to Jerne, the immune system is largely (98 percent) made up of small lymphocytes that can respond to an enormous variety of signals. Unlike the nervous system, they do not need to be connected by fibers because they can move freely about the body, interacting by direct encounter or by the antibody molecules that they release. As they recognize and are recognized, they modulate themselves, adapting to the outside world, learning from experience, and building up a memory that is sustained by reinforcement and can be deposited in lasting network modifications (Jerne 1974:377, 387). In an effort to capture the tremendous information capacity of the immune system and its responsiveness to alterations of its environment, it is sometimes called a "mobile brain" (Endroczi 1989).

Some researchers have drawn out an important implication from Jerne's view: the immune system is not composed of "self" poised and ready to attack any "nonself" that ventures into "self" territory. It is not, as in the usually accepted view, "ignorant" or "tolerant" of "self" (hence not attacking self) and knowledgeable about or responsive only to nonself. Instead, what the immune system does is maintain the organization of itself. Foreign materials can be "seen" by the immune system only in the form of "internal images" of them; because of the infinite variety of antibodies produced by somatic mutation, all possible varieties of the foreign have already been made in advance. Hence, the immune system sees only self, knows only self (see fig. 21): "The system has no way (and no need) of distinguishing self from foreign. It knows nothing alien to its composition. It only knows of itself, and its self is the network of endogenous activity." This approach moves from a paradigm of the immune system not seeing the self (lest it attack) to a paradigm of the immune system not seeing the foreign. By means of somatic mutation, it has already anticipated, inside "self," every variety of the "nonself" that it could ever meet. It is not that the immune system never has an important antimicrobial defense role but that "the system is more than a sophisticated biological warfare machine" (Coutinho et al. 1984:153–54, 155).

Although most immunologists treat these ideas with skepticism ("Networks" 1991:154), a recent issue of *Immunology Today* devoted its main review section to two articles presenting new data on the "metadynamical plasticity of immune networks" (Avrameas 1991; Varela and Coutinho 1991). In time it may be that a model of the immune system as a complex regulatory system will be accepted: as the editors of *Immunology Today* (May 1991, iii) say, it is possible that "regulatory principles, in the form of regulatory networks, emerge spontaneously from the complex cellular and molecular interactions of the immune system."

Just as we found in Chapter 2 that nonscientists in the larger society hardly ignore the immune system in their understanding of health, so in this chapter we find that immunologists and scientists interested in immunology do not ignore the world outside the lab in devising their models of the body. Is immunology more open at its borders than other fields in biology? In their willingness to consider unconventional organizing ideas, the many scientists to whom we talked suggested that this was so. Is immunology's openness as a field related to its reliance, since the dramatic changes of the 1970s, on a model of the body as a complex system that is in constant, anticipatory, flexibly adaptive change? Or is it related to the amount of change that the field's body of knowledge has experienced under the impetus of AIDS and many other factors, something many scientists we interviewed described as "dramatic" or "explosive"?

Whatever the answer to these speculative questions, one conclusion emerges clearly from the explorations in this part of the book. The views on the immune system of the nonscientists in Chapter 2, the alternative practitioners in Chapter 3, and the scientists in Chapter 4 are all closer to each other than the images used by the media seen in Chapter 1. Thus, we would do well to be cautious in taking the content

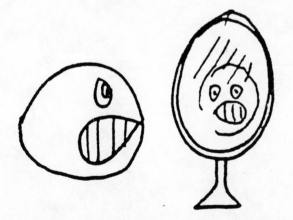

Fig. 21. *Umberto Eco's "doodle" of an immune system cell looking into a mirror and "seeing self." From E. E. Sercarz et al., eds.,* The Semiotics of Cellular Communication in the Immune System *(1988:171).*

of the media as symptomatic of what is thought to be known in the society about the body, health, and the immune system. It also means that "science," even the biological sciences, cannot be taken to be a unitary field of knowledge, given that differences in basic operating assumptions exist among specialties.[9]

Strange but wonderful bedfellows can emerge from ethnographic inquiry into knowledge about the body, allowing us to enjoy the meeting of the minds between Vera Michaels, who imagined the immune system as "the waves," evoking a turbulent, chaotic phenomenon in constant change; Patricia O'Hara, the acupuncturist who saw the healthy body as "rivers flowing without interruption, without being dammed up"; and Bruce Kleiner, a research scientist who wondered whether T cells could be traversing the depths of tissues to "whisper in the ears of neurons."

PART
FOUR

CONFIGURATIONS OF HEALTHY BODIES

CONFIGURATION: *arrangement of parts or elements in a particular form or figure; the form, shape, figure, resulting from such arrangement; conformation, outline, contour. 1936 R. Linton Study of Man: The function of a trait complex is the sum total of its contribution toward the perpetuation of the social-cultural configuration.* COMPUTING: *The way the constituent parts of a computer system are chosen or interconnected in order to suit it for a particular task or use.*

The Oxford English Dictionary

CHAPTER 5

Complex Systems

New surges of life are pounding at circumference and centre; we must open the way for their entrance and onflow. To-day the individual is submerged, smothered, choked by the crowd fallacy, the herd theory. Free him from these, release his energies, and he with all other Freemen will work out quick, flexible, constantly changing forms which shall respond sensitively to every need.

MARY PARKER FOLLETT, *The New State*

A re people really coming to think of their bodies as complex systems embedded in other complex systems? What is a *complex* system?[1] What are the implications of applying a systems model to the body and health for our sense of our selves and our ability to change the world?

To begin answering these questions, we need an ethnographic description of how systems models work in daily life. One thing makes such a description particularly tricky: systems models are currently being used as descriptive devices throughout the physical sciences, social sciences, and humanities, perhaps because they seem to capture best the actual nature of the world in which we live at the end of the twentieth century. My task will be to describe the main features of a complex systems model while keeping open the question of the extent to which the model "fits" the world.

For a taste of what complex systems theory (also called *chaos theory* or *nonlinear dynamics*) is like and an example of how it has been used by an ethnographer to describe his field site, I turn to the work of Antonio Benitez-Rojo.[2] In his ethnography of the Caribbean, he argues that it is a field

> quite in tune with the objectives of Chaos. . . . Within the (dis)order that swarms around what we already know of as Nature, it is possible to observe dynamic states or regularities that repeat themselves globally. . . . Chaos looks toward everything that repeats, reproduces, grows, decays, unfolds, flows, spins, vibrates, seethes; it is as interested in the evolution of the solar system as in the stock market's crashes, as involved in cardiac arrhythmia as in the novel or in myth. Thus chaos provides a space in which the pure sciences connect with the social sciences, and both of them connect with art and the cultural tradition. . . . I have tried to analyze certain aspects of the Caribbean while under the influence of this attitude, whose end is not to find results, but processes, dynamics, and rhythms that show themselves within the marginal, the regional, the incoherent, the heterogeneous, or, if you like, the unpredictable that coexists with us in our everyday world. (Benitez-Rojo 1992:2–3)

Within biology, but far afield from the immune system, ecologists explain how "populations of certain grasses, following an internal dynamic, rise and fall in the irregular, unpredictable patterns that scientists call chaos." "Ecologists are increasingly abandoning the popular concept of the balance of nature and are replacing it with the image of a natural world in which plant and animal communities perpetually fluctuate. Disturbances like climatic change, fires, storms, and disease, some scientists say, seldom give these communities the chance to settle into a state of equilibrium" (Stevens 1991:4).[3]

In our interviews, among the many captivating ways in which people develop the notion of a complex system, a few descriptions stand out because they clearly contrast complex systems with mechanical systems.[4] A biologist holding a position as a postdoctoral fellow explains the shift from looking at the "nuts and bolts" in the machinery of the body to looking at how the nuts and bolts function when they are embedded in complex systems:

A lot of the concepts that looked pretty simple, now [are] looking much more complicated. That's on the one hand. On the other hand, the other aspect that I like about immunology is that it's a science of systems, of interacting systems. And I always like interacting systems, which is the thermodynamic aspect of systems. So it's a system which had many, many elements. Many, many specificities of antibodies. Many, many types of cells interacting in many, many ways. . . . The new vision of the new thermodynamics of open systems will be interesting. Once we have all the nuts and bolts together, we'll be able to look at it as a system, and understand what's underneath. (Ken Holden)

A medical school student reflects on the implications of using different sorts of imagery to explain illnesses to patients. He acknowledges that he has been schooled to think of antibodies in terms of the traditional militaristic and violent imagery. Then he wonders whether patients' perceptions would be any different if doctors explained disease in a different way. He contrasts the military conflict model with another model: "You are interacting with the environment on a kind of more interface level . . . you are part of an environment and this is what's happening to you" (Allan Chase).

A health service administrator acknowledges that she typically thinks of the immune system in "violent" terms: "You do think of it as something that's alien to yourself, a germ, you know, a virus or a bacteria or something like that, you know, that's an alien, a little alien, kind of creeping in, and your body is going to get ready to defend itself and destroy the bad stuff, the bad guys" (Becky Randall). Would she necessarily have to think of it that way?

Well, just from your having asked that, I kind of realize that was the way I was looking at it. Now of course, the kind of intriguing part of the whole thing is that you can look at a lot of things that way. Or you can look at the viruses as being neither good nor bad. They have evolved a way of getting along, and it may not be very pleasant for us, 'cause they may give us a cold or something like that, but they evolve to do what they can in their environment, and they just do it until something happens, which is neither good nor bad, it's just that we don't like it very much.

With an easy fluency, she shifts from the point of view of her body, which, if victorious, will obliterate the "virus-other," to the point of view of the "other" that coexists, however uneasily, in her body.

WITH THIS BRIEF INTRODUCTION, let me present some of the features that characterize a complex system, setting it apart from either a simple system or a mechanical model.

Field Concept. The notion of a field underlies and makes possible the development of models of complex systems. It implies that "reality consists not of discrete objects located in space but rather of an underlying field whose interactions *produce* both objects and space. It further implies . . . that there is no exterior, objective viewpoint from which to observe, for one is always already within the field, caught in and constituted through the very interactions that one is trying to describe" (Hayles 1990:xi–xii).

Regulation. In the words of one of the founders of systems theory, Ludwig von Bertalanffy, we are in the midst of the Second Industrial Revolution, which involves control engineering: machines have regulatory circuits that provide them with explicitly goal-directed characteristics. "It is thus easily understandable," Bertalanffy writes, "that our present generation tries to interpret an organism as a complex regulatory mechanism while the seventeenth, eighteenth, and nineteenth centuries conceived it as a clockwork or a heat engine." He continues:

> The living organism . . . is a prototype of the Heraclitean *panta rhei*, maintaining itself in a continuous flow and change of components. The structures controlling the processes within the system itself are at the same time maintained and destroyed, amalgamated and regenerated, decomposed and recomposed. Modern scientific research has shown that this "dying and becoming" in an organism is taking place at an unsuspected speed. Principles guaranteeing the maintenance of a system in a continuous flow of its components, therefore, must be deeper than the widespread principle of regulation by means of feedback mechanisms. Do we know of any theoretical concepts or models

which can account for this situation? . . . The starting point is the concept of *open systems*. (Bertalanffy 1975:119; see also Hayles 1990:14)

In a discussion of the role played by systems thinking in the development of the atom bomb at Los Alamos, William Arney explains the role of regulation and control in the difference between simple and complex systems:

> Simple (goal-directed, single-loop, negative-feedback) systems have a certain continuity of action. Effect follows cause until the system monitoring devices force the cause, through their *negative* feedback, to be removed or attenuated. When the cause is removed, the effect ceases. Complex systems sometimes behave discontinuously. Systems simply change states. In models of complex systems, a controlling loop may reach a threshold state and transfer control to another loop altogether. The system appears to have experienced a discontinuous jump from one set of apparent relationships dominating the action to another. (1991:51)

Nonlinearity. As Katherine Hayles explains this, "With linear equations, the magnitudes of cause and effect generally correspond. Small causes give rise to small effects, large causes to large effects. Linearity connotes this kind of proportionality. Equations that demonstrate it can be mapped as straight lines or planes. Nonlinear functions, by contrast, connote an often startling incongruity between cause and effect, so that a small cause can give rise to a large effect" (1990:11). This feature is closely related to the one to which I turn next.

Sensitivity to Initial Conditions. In models of weather systems, this is often called "the butterfly effect," after the notion that a butterfly beating its wings in Brazil today could set off tornadoes in Texas tomorrow (Kellert 1993:12; Gleick 1987:8). In complex systems, tiny differences in input can lead to huge differences in output; in other words, complex systems are extremely sensitive to fluctuation and change.[5]

WHEN, during our fieldwork, people described the body as a complex system, they would often rely on some of the defining features that we have identified. A naturopathic pharmacist explains how his assumption that health results from the body's constantly changing states affects his prescriptions, emphasizing the concepts of regulation and nonlinearity within the body:

> What I'm discovering working with different medicinal plants, working particularly with acupuncture, is our body is a natural pharmacy. It's like a factory. Even when we give an antibiotic, it's not the antibiotic but our body's response that is making the effect. So if we can make [things] available to replenish that internal pharmacy and still stimulate the proper internal functioning . . . you're not forcing the body into one, two, or three responses. You're letting it pick and choose what it wants to do. *And the way it wants to do it?*
> The way it wants to do it. (Barry Folsom)

Here, Barry Folsom is using a quintessential image from the earlier, Fordist, era, the body as factory, but giving it functions suitable to an era of flexible specialization: flexibly and responsively, the body chooses what it wants to do when it wants to do it.

We also came across the term *vibrancy* used to describe the body as a complex system embedded in its environment. Discussing the view that parasites share a common environment with their human hosts, an immunologist describes this coexistence as a "vibrant spectacle." Moving easily from the part of the system that is human to that which is parasite, he comments, "A parasite that lives with you for fifty years is happy, but if it can infect your family, it's even happier" (Ron Wilder).

A minister whose parish is in an inner-city neighborhood has developed a highly articulated way of explaining the body as a system with vibrancy. In his view, vibrancy happens when his system works well and "moves," when it builds up energy and vigor, rather than when it has to expend energy defending its borders, fighting off invaders:

> I'd rather think about my system working toward building me up or keeping everything working well or functioning well, so that there's a lot of vibrancy. If my system has to spend a lot of time fighting off invaders, that is using a lot of energy that I would rather go into kind of maintaining vibrancy. . . . I also understand that there's a lot of invaders around, you know, and if they need to be fought off, they need to be fought off. There's not much you can do about it. You know, guys are doing their job then.

What do you mean about vibrancy?
General vitality. You know, I guess good to be alive, I can handle what comes along, I can have enough energy to do what is required of me in this day and to give what needs to be given, or at least offer it to other people. . . . I would rather think about my system, you know, working together for personal strength and vigor, and energy, brightness, that kind of thing. If it is that I have to spend a lot of inner strength fighting things off, that's just like if a group has to spend all of its time dealing with disagreements and dissensions and all like that. It maintains itself, but it tends not to move anywhere. I would rather think of myself as a system that doesn't have to do all that maintenance all the time, but it's a tough environment around here, you know, in terms of bacteria and stuff floating around. And so that has to happen. (Joe Elliott)

Joe Elliott regrets the necessity that his body at times has to defend its borders instead of building its vibrancy. Other people see the enterprise of defending borders as a fruitless one, given that the borders cannot be fixed; they see themselves as persons or bodies in a system with no clear, stable borders within it and no place outside it on which to stand. In thus articulating aspects of the field concept, people frequently make creative use of analogies to recent wars, which have complicated our simple notions of who is friend and who is foe, which is safe territory and which dangerous. Harry Wilson sees a similarity between the lack of borders in the Vietnam War and the lack of borders in the fight against AIDS:

See, we have to keep in mind, regardless of what you did over there, whether you were a cook, a door gunner, a pilot, a grunt, a radio man, a cook, a typist, you could still get killed any minute because it was no fun in Vietnam. Like you saw the fronts of World War I, World War II, trenches. . . . You see all these Vietnam War movies. Yeah, there were a small percentage of what they call *firefights*, between NVA or Vietcong and Americans, but not like you see on the TV. They boost it up.
There are no borders really?
No borders whatsoever. I was in Saigon many times, and I saw a girl sixteen or seventeen years old being at the wrong place at the wrong time. A Vietnamese girl was riding a moped, and I

guess someone had thrown a live charge into this bar. Well, unfortunately, she was in the path, so it hit her and just blew her right in half, forced her right in half, and you see a small, young girl, eighteen, ninteen, whatever, lying there blown in half. Or you know, you just see people along the road, lying around dead, or just burnt up, or mutilated, or whatever. I mean it was like hell. . . . There was no front, there was no front line. Yeah, my personal opinion, I don't think there's any front line in the war with AIDS. I mean, people say that blacks started it. No, I can't say it's the blacks. . . . No, I think it's any-where, black, yellow, red, green. I don't think there's any partic-ular color. (Harry Wilson)

Similarly, the Gulf War is used as an example of a war without clear borders. Mike Alvin, a scientist, grapples with what imagery will best capture the nature of immunological events. He prefers cops and rob-bers over warfare as a metaphor because it allows for the idea of call-ing for backup and infiltrating the "foreign" guys. To this extent he wants the sharp lines of the self/nonself distinction blurred. The rea-son he finds warfare inadequate as a metaphor for the immune system is that the nature of war has changed. You can no longer say who is the bad guy. Even in the Gulf War, Saddam was not the bad guy: "He had his purposes too." If you wanted to pick a war in which it was clear who was right, "which war would you pick?"

WHAT ARE some of the possible or likely consequences of thinking of the body as a complex system? The first consequence might be described as the paradox of feeling responsible for everything and pow-erless at the same time, a kind of empowered powerlessness. Imagine a person who has learned to feel at least partially responsible for her own health, who feels that personal habits like eating and exercise are things that directly affect her health and are entirely within her con-trol. Now imagine such a person gradually coming to believe that wider and wider circles of her existence — her family relationships, commu-nity activities, work situation — are also directly related to personal health. Once the process of linking a complex system to other complex systems begins, there is no reason, logically speaking, to stop. This cos-mic view of the body is the kind of thing that people are trying to express in comments like the following:

I think the healing model is really an inclusive model. As you move, instead of moving down the reductionistic path, they move up the holistic path . . . the integrated path. Each aspect that has a larger systemic nature to it incorporates everything below it. The cell is going to incorporate electrons and microbiology. The tissue is going to . . . and so on, and so on. So you begin to look at it from a cosmic consciousness point of view. You're really incorporating the whole thing. (Peter Boswell)

A farmer in New Jersey is going to be in some way, shape, or form related to a farmer in Des Moines. I mean I believe that. We're all related, everything, and not just people but the environment and the world and everything. It's all interrelated. I guess you could say it would be more of a Hindu concept that I believe. But I think, I even see that Jesus taught that. So I see everything as interrelated. You can't do one thing without it relating or affecting everything else in the system. Everything else changes. (Ned Germane)

If you see everything about your health connected to everything that exists but also accept the possibility of managing and controlling at least some of the factors, the enormity of the "management" task, of controlling one's body and health, becomes overwhelming. Who will manage all this? Is anyone in control? These are questions that give form to anxieties expressed in many of the interviews. A student in a college biology class reflects on the effect of seeing electron micrographs of cells inside the body:

I could think, like, *I have more control* because, you know, there are things you can do to affect something that's going on in your body, but then you think you could be in less control because there's so many other things in your body that, maybe, you don't know about. And they just go on constantly without even you thinking about them. So that I guess that could make you think that *I was, like, in less control, too*. A whole other world. (Martha Novick)

A hairdresser expresses vividly how complicated it is to manage the enormous amount of information that relates to her health:

I still think people need to have responsibility for their own health, and yet I can see that there's just so much that I don't know. You know, so much information, so much going on that I have no way of knowing, I can understand why it becomes so complicated, and it's not simple. . . . Cigarettes, for instance, they're saying people shouldn't smoke cigarettes. That's a good example, but, on the other hand, I don't think that cigarettes are this big evil enemy. I think there are probably some people that should never smoke a cigarette because they have, you know, a weakness in that area. There are people that can smoke their whole lives, and it doesn't seem to affect [them]. I don't know. I don't know. I just don't think things are that black and white. (Anita Higden)

An M.D. promulgates both the view that the systems affecting health are far too complex to be controlled by anyone and the view that people are responsible for their own health, even though they may feel guilty because they cannot control it:

So the body does have a natural life of its own, which the yogis are very clear to state. And there are ways which we can affect [it] and ways we can't. We can't stop aging, we can't stop death, we can't stop a lot of things. And so there are things we have control over and certain phases in our development that we do. . . . It's a new age perspective that's been very destructive for a lot of people with sickness 'cause it creates a lot of guilt around what I did or I didn't do — that's just insane. *Life is more complex than I can control it.* . . . There is far more capacity to self-regulate the physiological functions of the body than people imagined thirty or forty or fifty years ago. There's really enormous control that can be observed, much of which has been demonstrated through biofeedback. . . . So there's almost a re-owning of our own capacity to know our body, to experience it, to self-regulate it, to train it. (Peter Boswell)

Another consequence of viewing the body as a complex system is brought out vividly by William Arney in his discussion about the development of the atom bomb. In Arney's view, a sense of inexorability or relentlessness is brought about in complex systems. They are impervious to being pushed in any particular direction by any particular agent, "relentlessly resilient to change, rapidly responsive to criticism and stable. . . . [They] sustain themselves in response to most assaults from their environments" (1991:3). A particularly chilling example of inexorability fostered by a complex systems view was expressed by Robert Oppenheimer, as he described why he and others worked to develop the atom bomb: "When you come right down to it the reason we did this job is because it was an organic necessity. If you are a scientist you cannot stop such a thing" (quoted in Arney 1991:113). The scientific expert in this situation is like an "agent of necessity, an executive of the inevitable. There is an irresistibility to the rationality that says it is but one's job to help something realize its potential" (Arney 1991:113). Like Oppenheimer, individuals lose a sense of agency in the face of the systemic forces that appear to be overwhelmingly and inexorably playing themselves out.

Because complex systems can be resilient in the face of change, they are closely associated with the dampening of conflict. Thus, a third consequence of systems models applied to the body is that conflict can come to seem unthinkable. Like simple systems, complex systems can handle discord (say, illness) in one part by making adjustments in another to return to a steady state of harmony (health) (Young 1985). We will see in later chapters that the health of the body and the corporate organization seen as systems seems to require a profound dampening of conflict between husbands and wives, parents and children, management and labor, men and women, whites and minorities.[6]

But the features of a complex system that make it different from a simple system can lead to a different outcome. Because control can suddenly shift from one part of the system to another, and because small initial causes can have large effects, health and harmony are by no means guaranteed. Instead, sudden, catastrophic eruption or collapse can, and indeed eventually *will*, occur.

The last consequence of seeing everything made up of systems within systems is that humans and human purposes are no longer considered preeminent, as they typically have been in Western humanistic traditions: "The systems world may be for humans, *but* it may not be. . . . Systems create a certain equivalence between humans and other subsystems of the global system and lead directly to the concept of substitutability among sub-systems. There is no priority of human living over any other sub-system within the global system. The sub-system of 'living human beings' is, from a systems perspective, conceptually equivalent to the 'waste management' sub-system, for example" (Arney

1991:57–58). This leads to a certain indifference to specifically human life, which inspires Arney to term this aspect of a systems perspective its "necrophilic" character.

A medical student thought about how he would explain the immune system to a class of high school students. Certainly without intending any callousness, he went on to illustrate vividly Arney's point about how systems thinking encourages an indifferent attitude toward distinctions among subsystems:

> I guess I'd like to use a less military kind of approach. I think that we're part of an environment. I think AIDS is an interesting disease because it . . . actually causes the boundaries of the human being to be blurred between self and environment. The things that can't [usually] grow in you can grow in you. . . . People become culture mediums. I mean, you become a substance upon which many things can grow, can grow and flourish. If you look at it from the microorganism's point of view, they can now grow and flourish in you. You become this kind of incredible rich ground upon which to multiply. I know that's disturbing from the human being's point of view. (Allan Chase)

My argument in this chapter comes to this: in the late twentieth century, complex systems models provide a pervasive way of thinking about the world, about our bodies, about our societies, and to think in these terms may have certain significant consequences. All too often, accounts of the world from a systems perspective argue, as do David Levin and George Solomon, that a systems view of the mind-body relation will "restore the body to the larger world-order" (1990:524) and overcome the shortcomings of mechanistic views of medicine and the body. As we will see in coming chapters, Arney's theoretical statements are too full of despair, and Levin and Solomon's too full of hope, adequately to capture the complicated ways in which people struggle to comprehend their bodies, in health and disease, as complex systems.

CHAPTER 6

System Breakdown: "Dying from Within"[1]

"This is the nature of modern death," Murray said. "It has a life independent of us. It is growing in prestige and dimension. It has a sweep it never had before. We study it objectively. We can predict its appearance, trace its path in the body. We can take cross-section pictures of it, tape its tremors and waves. We've never been so close to it, so familiar with its habits and attitudes. We know it intimately. But it continues to grow, to acquire breadth and scope, new outlets, new passages and means. The more we learn, the more it grows. Is this some law of physics? Every advance in knowledge and technique is matched by a new kind of death, a new strain. Death adapts, like a viral agent. Is it a law of nature? Or some private superstition of mine? I sense that the dead are closer to us than ever. I sense that we inhabit the same air as the dead. Remember Lao Tse. 'There is no difference between the quick and the dead. They are one channel of vitality.' He said this six hundred years before Christ. It is true once again, perhaps more than ever."

DON DELILLO, *White Noise*

Shortly after the eighth International Conference on AIDS in Amsterdam in the summer of 1992, several editorials written by scientists in science publications and many articles in the major printed news media appeared that cast doubt on some of the assumptions that had been guiding AIDS research for the last decade.[2]

The precipitating events at the conference were reports of about thirty people who had all the symptoms of AIDS but no trace of HIV in their bodies (Chase 1992). Although these people were not present at the conference, it was literally the existence of their bodies, which did not fit into existing understandings of AIDS, that disrupted the proceedings. Some media coverage of this event focused on the terrifying possibility that the patients were infected with a new retrovirus that cannot be detected by current blood-screening tests (Gladwell 1992b; Cimons 1992; Gorman 1992). Other media coverage focused on whether the cases of HIV– individuals with AIDS vindicate an unconventional theory, much vilified by the medical establishment, that has been promulgated by Peter Duesberg, Joseph Sonnabend, and others. In the conventional view, AIDS is an infectious disease caused by the microorganism HIV. In the unconventional view, HIV is not the sole necessary and sufficient cause of AIDS; other lifestyle factors, such as drug use, severely impair the immune system, allowing HIV and many other microbes a foothold (Fumento 1992; Heimoff 1992).[3] Some of this media coverage railed at the spectacle of scientists wrangling among themselves about the etiology of AIDS: not only will a house divided against itself find it difficult to develop cures for AIDS, but mixed messages about what causes AIDS (and therefore how to prevent it) will confuse the public (Heimoff 1992).

In science journals, the events at the conference were not construed so negatively. Naming what is going on as a "sea change" (Cohen 1992:153) or a change in the "current AIDS paradigm" (Sterling 1992:4), these professional science articles turned the attention of the general science community toward the deeply divided opinion within the AIDS research community about how the disease should be conceptualized.[4] Striking evidence of the division of opinion is found in the fact that about fifty scientists have formed the Group for the Scientific Reappraisal of the HIV/AIDS Hypothesis (Sterling 1992).

As *Science* explains the debate, in the view that has guided research since AIDS was first recognized, the human immunodeficiency virus (HIV) is taken to be the cause of AIDS. Even though a person infected with the virus might not show symptoms of illness for years, the assumption is that all those infected will eventually fall ill. A further assumption is that repeated exposure to the virus through sex is a virtual guarantee of infection (Cohen 1992:152). The contrary views draw attention to a great many anomalies that call the current paradigm into question. Among the anomalies are the following: some people who have been infected as long ago as the late 1970s remain asymptomatic; some people remain uninfected despite repeated exposure through sex (Cohen 1992:152); cases of AIDS have been diagnosed in people who test HIV–; some people who become infected with HIV subsequently lose all signs of infection, including seropositivity, and remain healthy (Root-Bernstein 1992:4).[5]

There are basically two alternatives to the current paradigm. The first questions how central or powerful the role of HIV is in causing AIDS. HIV infection may be a necessary but not sufficient condition (other factors such as drug use or malnutrition may need to be present to produce disease); HIV infection may be neither necessary nor sufficient (AIDS would then be a condition that could be caused by many immunosuppressive agents, of which HIV is only one) (Root-Bernstein 1992:5; Root-Bernstein 1993:27). The second view sees AIDS as an autoimmune disease in which HIV, perhaps with the help of other factors, tricks the body's immune system into attacking itself (JM 1991; Root-Bernstein 1992:5).

Both popular and scientific media agree that the implications of these shifts in how AIDS is conceived are dramatic. A *New York Times* editorial referred to AIDS research being "back to square one" (Kramer 1992). The cover of *Time* proclaimed that we are "losing the battle," and inside the magazine reported a "mood of despair" at the Amsterdam AIDS conference (Ungeheuer 1992:30). The *Utne Reader* concurred: "There's a growing sense that mainstream science has taken its best shot at AIDS — and missed. . . . The link between the human immunodeficiency virus (HIV) and AIDS may not be a simple case of cause and effect — the assumption that for eight years has been the basis for almost all AIDS research" (Creedon 1992:17). Newspapers reported that it is one thing to understand all about the virus but quite another to understand the immunologic basis of how the body responds to it. They quoted Jonathan Mann, the Harvard researcher who chaired the conference, as saying, "We are all working on the twigs, the leaves, the branches, but no one sees the forest," and Greg Gonsalves of the Treatment Action Group as saying, "There is a real lack of research on basic immunology. Nobody has the money to fund it" (Gladwell 1992a:26).

Instead of focusing on "correlates of [disease] progression," *Science* magazine reported that researchers will now start to look at "correlates of protection" (quoted in Cohen 1992:152). In other words, instead of looking at the activities of the viral agent, researchers will begin to try to understand how people who have the agent in them but are not sick, or ought to have the agent in them but do not, stay well. This means that attention shifts to how the immune systems of these people function as a whole *and* what their lives are like as a whole: "It is not just exposure to HIV that must be considered in determining risk for AIDS but the status of the immune system during and after HIV exposure. People who are healthy, or who adopt healthier life-styles after HIV infection, may successfully combat HIV" (Root-Bernstein 1993:55).

However little is now understood about the details of this approach, strong voices are asserting that the single-factor model of causation that dominated research on HIV ought not to be carried over into this new era. Bonnie Mathieson of the Division of AIDS, a branch of the National Institute of Allergy and Infectious Diseases, thinks that "the lesson to be learned here is that there may never be a single correlate of protection, be it antibodies or cell-mediated immunity. 'Everyone's looking for one correlate of immunity,' says Mathieson. 'In the end, that's not what it's going to be'" (Cohen 1992:154).

Since the eighth AIDS conference, it is frequently implied in the press that virologists will have to become immunologists to understand HIV. This is a way of saying that virologists will not be able to understand the tiny microbes that they study in isolation unless they understand them in the context of the immune system as a complex system.[6] Some AIDS researchers have gone even farther, suggesting that understanding AIDS as "caused by a single disease agent is invalid"; instead, it should be understood as a "multifactorial, synergistic disease" (Root-Bernstein 1993:104ff.) or, in the terms discussed in Chapter 5, as a disease of the body conceived as a complex system. As we have seen, the domains of microbiology and the popular media actually lag far behind the popular imagination in thinking of health and the body in terms of a complex system. In this respect, then, the science of AIDS is now moving in a direction that *has already been taken* by the many people who have for some time been thinking of the body as a complex system.

A complex systems model of the body has much potential for offering a compelling picture of what AIDS is. As we learned in Chapter 5, in complex systems, slight differences in initial conditions can have magnified effects, and such systems contain randomness and disorder within order. Because of this, they carry the ready possibility of catastrophic collapse. What order there is, is local, transient, emergent, like "a whirlpool appearing in the flow of a river, retaining its shape only for a relatively brief period and only at the expense of incessant metabolism and constant renewal of content" (Bauman 1992a:189). Charles

Perrow explains that complex systems may collapse catastrophically because the "coupling" or linkage among parts of the system becomes too tight:

> Most of the time we don't notice the inherent coupling in our world, because most of the time there are no failures, or the failures that occur do not interact. But all of a sudden, things that we did not realize could be linked . . . became linked. The system is suddenly more tightly coupled than we had realized. When we have interactive systems that are also tightly coupled, it is "normal" for them to have this kind of an accident [a catastrophic collapse], even though it is infrequent. It is normal not in the sense of being frequent or being expected — indeed neither is true. . . . It is normal in the sense that it is an inherent property of the system to occasionally experience this interaction. (1984:8)

It is in precisely these terms that some analysts have been describing what AIDS does to the human body and to the human population on earth. In Mirko Grmek's historical account, the coupling of medicine and modern technology is implicated in making the epidemic possible:

> Medicine contributed to the epidemic as much by rupturing the fragile pathocenosis, that is by suppressing competing diseases, as it did by facilitating the transmission of the infection, notably through new means of direct blood contact. Moreover, modern technology contributed to the intermingling of peoples and the liberalization of social mores, both important factors in the emergence and dissemination of AIDS. The present epidemic is the other side of the medal of progress, the unexpected cost of having tampered radically with the ecological equilibria of the ages. (Grmek 1990:xi)

In sociologist John Gagnon's (1990:30) account, the AIDS epidemic is compared specifically to a common contemporary example of complex system breakdown, the Three Mile Island reactor's collapse.

In our fieldwork, it was not uncommon to hear explanations of the AIDS epidemic in terms of a system collapse. A genetic engineer saw AIDS as "crippling" the system:

What is a crippled system? You have a mutant, there is a particular autoimmune disease, a genetic or immune disease, or you
get AIDS, or you get whatever — something. Now, you have crippled the system. Now, what do you need to reconstitute it? We
have no idea. OK? We have taken away part of the system. . . . To
be able to understand what is the perturbation on the system, you
have to understand the whole balance of the system, and
nobody's even attempting to do this now. (Ken Holden)

For many people, at least part of the special horror aroused by the
contemplation of AIDS is the horror of system breakdown, which
could be seen as the coming of a nightmarish, random disaster, the
more horrible because known beforehand to be an ever-present possibility:

Can you imagine what it's like to have AIDS?
When I do imagine it, it's just one of the most horrifying. . . .
When I imagine what it's like to have AIDS, I imagine dying
from within. Just dying from within. All over the body, just
dying, every single inch of the body dying from within. Within
every finger, within every inch. That's how I look at it, and just
shivering up and down.
Is that what people have told you that it is like?
No. No one's told me what it's like. I mean, I've seen and read a
lot, and you see in lots of people, AIDS sufferers on TV and
I've known a few, and that's what it looks like, and that's what it
made me feel like it would be from inside. All the way into your
heart and your mind and everything.
And that would be different from the cancer process?
Well, I think of AIDS as being much worse than cancer. When
I think of cancer, most often I'll think of it in a certain area. I'll
think of it as a skin cancer or stomach cancer or liver cancer or,
you know, melanoma or brain cancer or tumors, you know.
When I think about AIDS, I just think of a whole body that's
just being taken. (Janey Wilcox)

Causes of this breakdown of the whole body system can come from
many places within the larger systems in which we live. The epidemic
of immune system dysfunctions, of which AIDS is part (lupus, chronic
fatigue syndrome, asthma), is often seen as a result of harmful forces

affecting all our bodies: pesticides in our water and food, background radiation, environmental pollution of all sorts, vaccinations against infectious diseases. As one person put it:

> To me it's all systemic. You can't localize and say this pathology here doesn't affect there. To me it's all one. When you look at what is it that makes the immune system break down, well, there are so many co-factors now, and because we don't want to acknowledge how many co-factors there are, we're always missing the boat. We don't acknowledge the environmental impact. Slowly, we're starting to. We don't acknowledge the background radiation. We don't acknowledge our food supply. We don't acknowledge the breakup of the family. We don't acknowledge the lack of spiritual meaning in people's lives. I mean the bottom line is we don't acknowledge the loss of meaning in people's lives and what that does to the human being. To me the HIV virus is a signature of an already weakened immune system. (Rebecca Petrides)

What are the images that people use to describe the impact of AIDS on the immune system? Our fieldwork yielded startlingly graphic images of the devastation wrought by HIV, attempts to capture the total nature of the system breakdown that AIDS entails. The AIDS virus was thought of as alien slime or as an ax striking to the core of a tree trunk:

> [The immune cells] have been neutralized so they're not making any assaults. I don't know, it's terrible to think about. Because there's nothing to fight back. This like thing comes and consumes you. It's like one of those, I never watch those horror movies, but it's like some kind of creeping, oozing stuff that just comes and possesses you. (Judy Lockard)

> When the virus [HIV] attacks the body, it just finds the right place to attack. I think the body works with a whole series of chemical reactions that are guided by other chemical reactions, and it's just like a tree spreading out branches, and I think if you hit an early enough branch, you will eventually get to the trunk, and that will shut everything down. And probably you're hitting some little leaf at the very edge when you have a cold. That's just

one small little virus, but with something like AIDS, you're hitting the trunk, so that shuts [off] everything downstream. (Marsha Wilmslow)

Many years ago, the immunologist Paul Ehrlich wrote about "horror autotoxicus," "the horror of becoming toxic to yourself" (Silverstein 1989:162). Probably without benefit of having read about Ehrlich, some people also expressed horror at the idea of a system turning against itself. As we saw in the last chapter, when thinking in terms of complex systems, harmony is expected and conflict unthinkable. Nonetheless, these expectations perch on the edge of chaotic breakdown:

It's frightening. It's almost like you expect everything in your body to be working harmoniously. I guess it's the same deal with cancer somewhat, where something that you trust like your lungs suddenly turn against you, you know, grow out of control basically. I think the people that have a disease like that feel especially betrayed by their body. . . . I guess that the feeling would be betrayal first, you know. How can my immune system turn against me? You know? What have I done? (Michael Spicer)

As we saw earlier, people frequently see the body as a system embedded within other, wider systems. Construing AIDS as a form of system breakdown sometimes strongly implicates those wider systems, whose breakdown in turn can affect the body's susceptibility to AIDS:

AIDS is a total assault on the immune system. It relates to all about them [patients], including their relationships with others. (Allan Browner)

AIDS is a breakdown of the body's life force. (Anthony Humphreys)

When the immune system shuts down, this can be caused by low self-esteem, which in turn can be caused by abuse and discrimination against homosexuals in our society. (Frank Saviano)

The sign of disease, such as virus or bacteria, may be a product rather than a cause. The cause can be weakness of the person, of the spirit or the soul. (Laura Peterson)

Very much as cancer patients, like Susan Sontag (1978), sometimes reject views of their disease that blame the victim, those immediately threatened by HIV are often ambivalent about views of AIDS like these that can seek its causes in "weakness of the person." A woman who is a member of ACT UP is angered by the common supposition that you can control your health by positive self-images. Such a view blames us for HIV, she thinks, and plays on the ways in which we have already been trained to feel guilty (Mara Whitman).

But other people take very seriously the possibility that one's self-image could directly affect the course of one's infection. John Parker, who is worried about his HIV status, says that he will not be tested. He is afraid of the effect on his health if he tests positive. He believes that the despair that he expects he would feel over his coming suffering and death might affect his body's functions and make him likely to succumb quicker. Sometimes such beliefs can lead to disillusionment: Ron Chappell, who has had AIDS for many years, says that he used to think that he had greater power over his immune system than he does now. He went to a weekend workshop devoted to improving health through positive thinking and found that it did not help him.

As we saw in Chapter 5, thinking of the field of systems related to the body as a system can produce simultaneous feelings of empowerment and powerlessness. With respect to AIDS, people can simultaneously experience a sense of universal agency (Everything is related to this disease: I will fix everything!) and helplessness (If I can't fix everything, and who could, then I will die from this disease). Although this empowered powerlessness could certainly lead to anxiety or enervation even in someone who is completely healthy, it might cause more profound distress in someone with a serious illness such as AIDS. Once we start to see the healthy body as if it were a complex system teetering along the path of life pretty well most of the time but always on the verge of falling over the edge into catastrophe, a pervasive sense of anxiety that is difficult to assuage seems inevitable.

Do people see the system breakdown of AIDS as contagious? We encountered two primary responses to this. As one person told us, total breakdown of your internal system is like a broken leg: you can't catch the state of being broken from another person: "[AIDS is] a broken immune system that can't remember what to do. . . . It's within that other person, and it's not a germ that comes out of their mouth. [It's] something broken within that person. . . . [It's] more like a broken leg. You don't catch a broken leg" (Mary Loran).

But, because there is also a singularly lethal agent involved, HIV, that can leak through the orifices or porous borders of one's or someone else's body, people worry about the integrity of their own body systems. It is perhaps out of this worry that the older model of the body sealed tightly behind its defended borders can reemerge with great potency in certain contexts. The "body at war" can reemerge even in the midst of a prevailing complex systems model that constantly erodes the significance of body borders and emphasizes the interconnection of everything.[7]

When our study was near its beginning, we interviewed Mary Blackstone, who worked for the city school system. I remember being struck by her panic over whether she might catch AIDS as she worked. What worried her was that she had to "handle the public" and handle lots of paper. Handling the paper gave her paper cuts, and, fearful that handling the public would subject her to HIV infection through these cuts, she washed her hands many, many times during the day. I remember discussing in our weekly project meeting how unreasonable and hysterical her fear of HIV seemed.

But this happened before I became a buddy and before I had experienced fear of HIV infection myself. Taking care of my first buddy, Mark Scott, and occasionally helping take care of the other residents of his home involved contact with "body fluids" beyond anything I could have imagined. One of the other residents was Thomas Solloway, a twenty-year-old African-American man who had been about to graduate from college, where he had played varsity athletics, when he came down with AIDS. By the time I met him, he was skeletally thin and too weak to sit up, stand, or even turn over in bed without assistance. His mind was often confused, and his speech was so slurred that hardly anyone could understand what he was saying.

One day, Mildred Pullman, the home's day health worker, called up to me where I was visiting Mark in his room on the second floor to come quickly and help her. Thomas had defecated in his bed, and his thrashing efforts to deal with the mess had spread soft and sticky feces all over him, the sheets, the bedcovers, and the floor. Mildred wordlessly handed me a pair of surgical latex gloves as she put on a pair herself, looking at me grimly. Together we managed to carry Thomas into the bathroom and lower him into the tub, which she had filled with hot water. Mildred instructed me to wash him while she dealt with the bed. Holding Thomas with one arm to keep him sitting upright, I did my best to sponge him clean. The water started out hot and sudsy but rapidly turned brown as I washed him off, and in no time at all the water had liberally filled up the inside of my wrist-length latex gloves. There seemed no point in replacing these gloves until Thomas's bath was over.

Later, wearing a new pair of gloves, I found out how easily the gloves tear. Just gathering up Thomas's soiled linens and carrying them down to the washing machine was sufficient to produce a large hole in one of the gloves, which I did not notice until I was finished.

This was my first major exposure to bodily fluids that probably contained HIV, but there were to be many more. Handling Mark's urine, sputum, saliva, nasal mucus, tears, and blood were all daily parts of visiting him, and, as I got to know him better and better, it became harder and harder to wear protective gloves at all. Soon I was doing just what Mary Blackstone did, washing my hands all the time. The problem was that this exacerbated the deep cracks I get in my hands in the winter, the very cracks in my defenses through which I had already imagined contagion from Thomas in the bathtub.

By this time, I had a very different reaction to the things that people were saying about their fears of HIV in our interviews. I too had minor panic attacks, when I was sure that HIV had made its way through a paper cut or a crack in my dry skin. No amount of rational discussion with myself about risk factors, the presence of soap in the bathtub water, the fragility of HIV in air, etc. did anything at all to allay my anxiety. Whenever I got a sore throat, swollen glands, flu-like symptoms, or a fever, all normal parts of life in my household with two school-age children, I became convinced that I was in the early stages of HIV infection.

ALSO LIKE many people we interviewed, I was profoundly reluctant to be tested. When, after the research had gone on for two years, I needed to be tested in order to begin a project in the immunology lab (all lab workers who might contact human blood had to be tested before they began), I thought that I would have the test done as a matter of course. But, in fact, I carried the form requesting the test around in my purse for about six weeks until it simply fell apart.

I know that similar fears afflicted other volunteers. One told me about a panic attack she had when a part of her skirt accidentally dipped into the toilet bowl used by the HIV+ person she was visiting. Gay men who were HIV– living with partners who were also HIV– could also be afflicted by similar anxieties. One couple discussed their paranoia over contracting HIV from each other because, even though they had tested negative, the virus "could be lying dormant there" (Peter Black and Frank Wallace). Only partly joking at the extent of their fear, one of them commented, "I can't just be normal."

Outside intimate relations, circumstances that people encounter at work are filled with threat. A graphic designer worries whether someone might have cut a finger and left infected blood on the blade of an exacto knife in her office; lab technicians who work with human blood dress in protective gear "like going into battle" and worry about small cuts, bitten cuticles, any break in their skin. A police cadet fears infection by being bitten: she told us that, when a suspect is immobilized, he often regresses to more primitive behavior — like biting — in response to being powerless. An undertaker told us that it is simply impossible to observe "universal precautions" for all cadavers because of the increased time and expense entailed. Therefore, he faces risk and fear in all cases not explicitly known to have been HIV–.

Although the HIV hotline workers we interviewed stressed how they attempt to allay widespread fears that people have of catching HIV from unlikely sources (such as eating a salad prepared by a gay waiter who might have cut his hand and bled into it), I have to wonder how effective rational discussion of risk factors can be. In September 1992, when Magic Johnson announced his return to professional basketball after a one-season absence following the announcement of his HIV+ status, the news coverage was filled with testimony from medical doctors about the possible risk to players of contracting the HIV virus from him during a basketball game:

> When four professional sports team doctors were asked how they would guard Magic Johnson, each, after a short reflection, gave the same answer: "I'd give him a lot of room." They did not laugh. They were not joking. They did not want to go on the record. One of those doctors said that while the virus certainly cannot be transmitted by casual contact — like hugging — basketball is not simply a contact sport, casual or otherwise. It is a collision sport. People regularly smash into one another. Blood spills. (Berkow 1992:31)

When, a month later, Magic announced that he had changed his mind and decided to retire after all, fear that other players had of contagion from him clearly played an important role (Goldstein 1992).

Dwelling on the subject of contagion makes it seem that, in the face of AIDS, people are holding each other at a distance, cowering inside their skins. But, unlike forty years ago, when our skins were our armor against disease, skin no longer protects us. Fear of contagion, fear of harm from others, makes AIDS seem like a "dark presence" that spreads its shadow over all of ordinary life, threatening every moment with a catastrophic collapse (Goldstein 1991:18).

As an overall impression of the public response to AIDS, this would be a misleading message. The dominant impression from our fieldwork is that, in widely varying ways, people are able to treat the effects of HIV as a "blessing and a curse." A pediatrician gave us an overview of this point of view:

> I think it's a blessing and a curse, and I think it's a blessing like any illness in certain individuals in that it can be a wake-up call to you when one learns one's own sero status. A friend of mine recently was diagnosed with melanoma and is responding the same way. His life is different now. It's richer in a lot of ways. His priorities are in order — that's a blessing. There have been some blessings for science that will be applicable to other diseases, and I think that there've been some changes in society which have been good for society that all marginalized groups have started to work together a bit more effectively than they ever would have ordinarily. That people who ordinarily would never deal with a marginalized person, some of those people actually feel called to get involved in the epidemic, and that means that they have to work with gays, they have to work with black people, they have to work with you know, people they never would invite over for dinner, and that's a blessing. But it's a curse. I mean there's no reason for us at our ages to have to go through these developmental things that are appropriate for seventy-year-olds, you know. (Robert Davies)

Lisa Demarco muses on how the threat of HIV pulls everyone in the population together because it appears in an activity (sex) that is not optional for most people: "Now that it's reached the heterosexuals, I think there's more of a scare. Now it's not my friend who's the artist, now it's not my florist, now it's not my gardener, but it's my son, it's my sister, it's myself. Illness is the great unifier when things have broken down." Charles Kingsley elaborates on the potential breaching of categorical distinctions that can be brought about by a common threat to health and life:

> You know, it's like, whether you're straight or whether you're gay, or whether you're black or whether you're white, whether you're young, whether you're old, you're human. You're a human being, you're a person. You know? And when you're talking in terms of a disease that's killing people, it's killing people. It shouldn't make a fucking difference if they're gay or if they're straight or if they're black or if they're white. It's killing people. Let's get it together, and let's get it taken care of. You know? I have just as strong of a feeling that they need to find a cure for sickle cell anemia as I do for AIDS, or cancer, or any other disease that's affecting the human population.

For people whose lives are only tangentially touched by AIDS, statements like these about the complexity of AIDS as a blessing and a curse, about the fragile boundaries that protect against AIDS, or about the barriers that AIDS can break down may be deeply felt, but they can go only so far toward encompassing the experience of having AIDS. In *Local Knowledge*, Clifford Geertz described ethnography as moving from "the immediacies of one form of life to the metaphors of another" (1983b:48). I want to make the opposite move now, from theoretical speculations about what AIDS is or what it means to considering the experience of having AIDS as an immediate part of daily life. As anthropologist Susan DiGiacomo asks about literary analyses of the meaning of illness, "If your disease is only a figure of all that is corrupt, sinister, and deadly, what could your actual death signify?" As she asks other anthropologists who "have considered every imaginable vantage point from which to observe affliction except the view from the hospital bed" and who have therefore refused to number themselves among the sufferers, how can we relate our lived experience so that we convey what *matters* culturally about the experience of illness (DeGiacomo 1992:125, 111–12)?

One extraordinary fieldwork event made me realize how often most of us are positioned as "immune witnesses" to AIDS, however deep our involvement with the epidemic.[8] Unless we are infected with HIV, there comes a point when we, unlike those who are infected, can watch safely from the outside, even as we may grieve for those who are "dying from within." The event involved a couple, Harry Ross and Ron Chappell. Monica Schoch-Spana, who was there, and I both knew Ron and Harry through our common membership in more than one AIDS activist organization. During the interview, Harry, who has had AIDS for some time, used the tape recorder while Monica was out of the room to force Ron to face his (Harry's) impending death and to express his wish that Ron, who is HIV–, would want to join him in infection and death. (During this conversation, Harry was lying on the couch holding the tape recorder on his chest while he questioned Ron, sitting at the other end of the couch.)

HARRY: And what are your concerns about becoming infected by me?
RON: Well, that might happen.
HARRY: How and why are you concerned about it? How can you be concerned about it? [Monica returns]
RON: [To Monica.] You've got to tell him to turn the tape off.
MONICA: What's that?
RON: You have to make him turn the tape off.
HARRY: No, no I don't. Why are you not concerned —
RON: He's interrogating me.
MONICA: Using my equipment? Sorry, no way, Harry.
HARRY: [Eluding Monica's effort to get her tape recorder back.] This is a nonscientific experiment — [Laughs. Then says to Ron] Would you prefer to be infected by me, and then you could follow me to the grave?
RON: No.
HARRY: So therefore you're willing to live without me for the next fifty years?
RON: I don't know if I'm willing. I could, I don't want to die. I don't want to see you die.
HARRY: But you don't want to die ever?
RON: Well, I will die.
HARRY: Well, who's to say it's not tomorrow?
RON: No one.
HARRY: Well then why aren't you prepared?
RON: Why aren't I prepared to die?

HARRY: Uh huh. You've got high blood pressure, got high cholesterol, all kinds of these viruses running through your blood, and
you're not worried about being, I mean really, you've got a dog
that could bite you, rip apart your jugular vein, and I would
love to watch you bleed, because I want to touch you, because
it might be infected.
[Monica finally manages to get the tape recorder away from
Harry.]

Harry asserted earlier in the interview that "everything connects. I
am going to get something out of this." For Harry, facing the actuality
of his own death in an immediate sense, the extensive network of social
support that he has developed assures him that he will not die alone.
But he wants more: he wants Ron to be infected and die with him. This
is an almost unspeakable desire, one that Harry wanted to express and
record (partly for himself and partly for our research), and one that he
wanted to use to confront Ron. Ron cannot grant this desire of his
dying partner; he cannot even speak it as a wish. Harry thus reveals to
us the utter solitude of dying, even when surrounded by one's lover and
friends.

This extraordinary exchange speaks profoundly of the boundaries
beyond which most of us cannot possibly imagine crossing or asking
another to cross. It speaks of the limits of the differences that it is possible for almost any of us to overcome — perhaps unless we too already
feel that we possess the passport of death.

CHAPTER 7

Flexible Systems

> *The kid had play in him. The kid had* flex, *and flex was rare. Flex was intelligent, special, a good sign, like big paws on a puppy. For a minute Strike lost his anger, entranced by this kid, by possibilities.*
> RICHARD PRICE, *Clockers*

A key concept in systems theory, one that we have already seen at work in the ways in which immunologists like to talk about parts of the immune system, is *flexibility*. In this chapter, I want to pursue the dimensions of this concept, illustrating its use in a wide variety of domains in contemporary culture, and showing its pervasive role in visual images of many kinds. Looking at the notion of flexibility in many different contexts will show us the wider cultural meanings of a key term in scientific immunological discourse and deepen our understanding of why this notion is now regarded so positively.[1]

As we have seen, one of the central attributes of complex systems is that, unlike mechanical systems, they are never in equilibrium. Everything is in flux, continuously adjusting to change (Rifkin 1983:186). A part of the ability to adjust continuously to change is what has been called *loose coupling*. Compared to tightly coupled systems, loosely coupled ones contain more slack and allow more variation. They can make spur-of-the-moment changes, adjustments, and innovations, and they can flexibly incorporate shocks, failures, or pressures for change (Perrow 1984:92). Most examples of loosely coupled systems are taken from manufacturing or service organizations; other systems theorists suggest, however, that the human body itself is a good example of a loosely coupled system. Pagels argues that, if in our intellectual pursuits we could imitate the body, with its versatility, plasticity, endurance, and survivability, its sloppy fits and all, we would "be assured of the survivability and flexibility of our knowledge" (1989:269).

As we will see in more detail in Chapter 11, this bundle of ideas about flexibility has become central to a substantial movement in contemporary human resource management and, through this route, has had an enormous impact on the way in which many manufacturing and service industries are reorganizing themselves. This school of thought (which often goes under the unwieldy name of *total quality management*) recommends that organizations become "continuously improving" organizations or "learning organizations." Very much on the model of a loosely coupled system, such a flexible organization can respond quickly to changes in its environment and can initiate changes in innovative ways. The following section of Hewlett-Packard's organizational values as they appear in their vision statement conveys the centrality of flexibility:

> *We encourage flexibility and innovation.* We create a work environment which supports the diversity of our people and their ideas. We strive for overall objectives which are clearly stated and agreed upon, and allow people flexibility in working toward goals in ways which they help determine are best for the organization. HP people should personally accept responsibility and be encouraged to upgrade their skills and capabilities through ongoing training and development. This is especially important in a technical business where the rate of progress is rapid and where people are expected to adapt to change. (Hiam 1992:62)

A Manager's Guide to Globalization enjoins its readers: "*Flexibility.* . . . The management of a global corporate culture that is adaptable and capable of dealing with rapid changes in the environment requires managers who are extremely *flexible*. Flexibility allows managers to meet the needs of the organization and to constantly adjust to global and local demands through coordination and allocation of the organization's resources" (Rhinesmith 1993:29). On a more local level, a book constructed as a charter to lead American businesses to success in the twenty-first century enjoins "flexibility and creativity," which "will be more important for success than endurance and loyalty." "Within business units of large organizations and within small companies, the most valued employees will be those who are flexible and can perform a wide range of functions" (Boyett and Conn 1991:4).

A front-page section in the Sunday *Baltimore Sun* on "The Shrinking Workplace" reports that contemporary plants will have to change to continuous-line production in order to respond "quickly to fickle fashion" (Lewthwaite 1993). An "empowered," "jack-of-all-trades" worker in such a factory comments about what's important: "Being flexible, being able to go from here to there and take care of whatever needs to be taken care of. I think if we all do that, we won't have a problem meeting the numbers" (p. 8A). Similarly, in the list of traits necessary for a successful manufacturing firm in *The Vest-Pocket CEO*, flexibility is central. Flexibility lies at the heart of the continuously changing, responsive organization (Hiam 1990:87).

It is important not to miss the tense dichotomy in the ways in which flexibility can be used by and in reference to organizations. On the one hand, as in the Hewlett-Packard value statement quoted above, it can mean something like freedom to initiate action: people set goals as they think best for the organization. (Of course, this depends on goal setting not being tightly controlled from above, a matter that the Hewlett-Packard statement leaves ambiguous.) On the other hand, it can mean the organization's ability to hire or fire workers at will, as in "Schools to Send Layoff Notices for 'Flexibility,'" which describes how twenty-one hundred employees in Los Angeles were to be laid off (Merl 1991). In this case, flexibility resides in the *schools*, and the employees have little choice but to comply. The powerful school system flexibly contracts or expands; the powerless employee flexibly complies.[2]

Laid-off workers are often enjoined to "stay flexible" if they want to regain employment (Whittingham-Barnes 1993). Often, the good, flexible worker is described as "nimble," as in the editorial "In Clinton's

Brave New World, Jobs for the Nimble," which pictures a group of workers frantically trying to leap out of the way of a hole being sawed in the floor under them (Neikirk 1992).[3]

A similar tension pervades an account of the "virtual office": "For years now, office workers have been begging for flexible time and the right to work at home. Now, more and more employers are saying yes, but for their own reasons. Companies committing themselves to the virtual office are practically pushing their employees out the door and into cars and spaces designed like hotels for drop-in work." Brought into being on the crest of "the business world's emphasis on flexibility in the work force," the virtual office is, in the words of one person who helps implement plans for them, "a way to create architecture and structure that can be so nimble and fast that we can stay ahead of change." But, like the nimble workers in "Clinton's Brave New World," workers in the virtual office are frightened for their jobs: "Fearful employees across the country, viewing trends toward 'downsizing,' part-time work and greater use of freelancers, tend to connect the virtual office with the virtual work force" (Patton 1993:C1, C6).

The tension between the highly desirable side of flexibility — activity, innovation — and the less desirable side — passivity, acquiescence — was painfully apparent in a discussion of the composition of the Clinton cabinet on PBS's "MacNeil/Lehrer Newshour." Representatives of women's groups, labor unions, and civil rights groups clashed with Joe Klein, senior editor of *Newsweek*. Klein had stated that groups like these have become anachronistic and reactionary: "We're in a new era now of governance, postmodern era when, you know, centralized bureaucracies are becoming anachronistic." Representatives of the "anachronistic groups" met these charges with outrage: women's rights or civil rights groups are not offering "rigid" solutions to problems; labor unions have actually demonstrated "great flexibility" over the last sixteen or more years. Unfortunately, the "flexibility" demonstrated by labor unions and civil rights groups during the Reagan-Bush years was often the flexibility of pliancy.[4]

Another complication concealed by the desirable aspects of flexibility is that workers who gain flexibility in their jobs may end up having to give up security. In a letter to the editor, a man reports that, as a freelance artist, he had to be able to devote his full attention to any assignment at a moment's notice. Hence, working for a temporary employment agency supplied just what he needed: "flexibility." However, he says, "if I could somehow forgo my need for flexibility, I would no longer wish to work as a temp." In his case, flexibility entails working without health insurance, paid vacations, paid sick days, bonuses, opportunity for advancement, and representation within the workplace. In short, "working without support and without a safety net within the corporate caste system, can be insufferable" (Hoppa 1993:16).

For an organization to capture the cachet of active, innovative flexibility, it helps to be entrepreneurial, engaged in market-oriented practices. More than one of our interviewees explained this to us, but none more clearly than John Blanchard, who works for an environmental protection organization:

> The state is more or less ossified. . . . It has absolutely no flexibility whatsoever. It does not respond to your needs as a consumer of state goods, of social goods, in any particularly comprehensive way. The marketplace, on the other hand, has the advantage of responding to your needs in that sense as flexibility 'cause it's a consumer marketplace. Response to demand and so on. . . . The state therefore becomes more and more ossified, you know. It's a cycle. The state just feels more and more rigid in what it can provide and what it can't provide.

The contrast between a rigid structure, its parts held in place in an inflexible way, and a loose structure, its parts able to move and change flexibly, is often taken to go along with a contrast between hostility and combativeness, on the one hand, and harmony and peace, on the other. For one example of how this notion has made its way into the larger culture, recent changes have taken place in the home design and construction industries, which in the past were "fraught with intractable formulas and phobias, stubborn codes and taboos" (Flanagan 1993). Faced with adversity, these industries are "becoming more responsive" in order "to survive" and are ready to "re-choreograph the three-way tango" between designer, builder, and client. In these shifting relationships, the emphasis is on flexibility. As a member of a design group summarized it: "The whole idea, which has a tremendous amount of flexibility, is for all three parties to cooperate and share information" (Flanagan 1993:1). The illustration accompanying this article shows graphically the harmony and cooperation that is to result from the rechoreographed singing and dancing of the designer, builder, and client (see fig. 22).

Architect to Client: 'Let's Work Together'

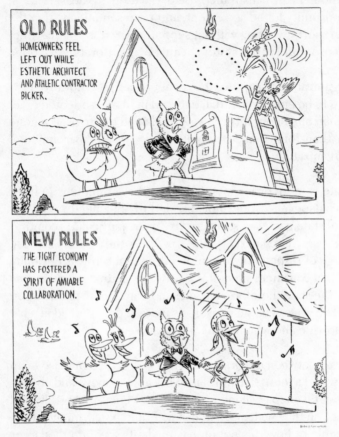

Fig. 22. *The transformation between old-style combative separation and new-style flexible cooperation in the home design and construction industries. From B. Flanagan, "Architect to Client: 'Let's Work Together,'"* New York Times, *13 May 1993, C1.*

To capture flexibility, it also helps to be small and nimble, like an elf. *Fortune* asks, "Is Big Still Good?" The answer, "Not necessarily. If giant companies are to survive, they must combine the benefits of size — lots of money, top talent — with the nimbleness of elves." The successful organization of tomorrow will consist of many small, decentralized units, "each with a laserlike focus on a market or a customer." The ideal is a "big organization that thinks flexibly" (Dumaine 1992:50, 51). We seem to be a long way from the immunology lab here, but in these very different contexts we again hear fascination with a certain kind of complex system, one that combines exquisite specificity with immense flexibility.

Flexibility in a system and its parts is increasingly seen as intrinsically valuable. As one indication of this, the word, often truncated as *flex*, is being applied to a plethora of products, companies, designs, and processes. Here is a selection mentioned in major newspapers over the last seven years:[5]

> *Products*. *FlexiGraphs*, including Flexibar and Flexispread, a type of presentation software; *Flexion*, a new jump rope; *FlexiTrace*, data acquisition software; *Flex-a-sizer*, a rod to strengthen and stretch muscles, *Tyrolia Free Flex*, a new ski binding; *Pro Flex*, wrist supports for repetitive-motion jobs; *Nordic Flex Gold*, a home exercise machine; *Flexeril*, a muscle relaxant; *FlexFile*, a labeling system.
>
> *Companies*. *Flex-n-gate*, a car parts company; *Petroflex*, a rubber manufacturer; *Flexi-van*, a truck lease and rental company; *Flex Products*, manufacturers of packaging that disintegrates in soil; *Flexible Interconnections*, and *Flextronics*, both electronic components manufacturers; *Flexible Bond, Inc.*, securities.
>
> *Designs*. *Flex* buildings; *flex* space, in which tenants can carry out multiple operations (warehouse, assembly, research, design, office work); *flexible factory*, in which the same production line turns out different products.
>
> *Processes*. *Flex plans*, flexible benefit plans; *flexography*, a method of printing newspapers on lighter paper; *flex time*, adjustable working hours; *flexiplace*, where technology allows workers to roam or work at home; *flexible weapons*, a sinister synonym for hand-to-hand fighting.[6]

Accompanying this multitude of uses of the concept of flexibility are many visual images intended to express its desirability. From personal finance to personal footware for one's self or one's children, flexibility is used to sell products. From Olsten's trademarked "the flexible workforce" to human resource management's "flexibility: the most important leadership tool of this decade," flexibility is used to sell services (see figs. 23–29).

The intense desirability — even the seductiveness — of the ability to be flexible and adaptive while in constant change is registered by the simultaneous appearance of this cluster of attributes in an exceedingly wide variety of domains. As far as I know, none of these areas could be claimed to be the single source for any or all of the others:

Immunology. As we saw in Chapter 4, antibodies, key elements in immunology's map of the body, are characterized by a combination of flexibility and specificity. In his essay for the *Encyclopedia Britannica*, Michael Edidin stresses the flexibility of antibodies, their "exquisite specificity," and sees the cells of the immune system engaged in an intricate "dance" (1991:24, 25, 37, 41). In immunology more generally, as more and more research is done, antibodies are looking more and more flexible. In addition to the variability of their overall shape through somatic mutation and the flexibility of their two arms, it now turns out that the binding site for the antigen itself (the socket in the ends of the arms) is also flexible. The fit between antigen and the binding site of the antibody is coming to be understood as an "induced fit" rather than a "lock and key" fit (Bhat et al. 1990). Rather than the precise but rigid specificity of a 1950s machine-tooled part, the binding site is coming to have the specificity of a 1990s flexible component, adjustable within limits to a variety of different environments.[7]

Computer Software. Computer programmers who worry about infection of their software by computer viruses often use basic immune system imagery to talk about how to handle the problem (Markoff 1992). To guarantee a "vaccinated" work station or a "sterilized" network, software vendors market products like "Vaccinate," "Disk Defender," or "Flu Shot +" (Ross 1991:79; Spanbauer 1993). They strive to have the operating system be based not on one model but on several diverse and flexible ones that can outsmart computer viruses by evolving faster than they do. Someday, it is hoped, each computer will be a slightly different variant of the standard and constitute a slowly evolving, flexibly adaptive "species" (Helmreich 1992; Kelly 1991:18–19).

Economics. Here the concept of flexible specialization, which first appeared in *The Second Industrial Divide* in 1984 (Piore and Sabel), is common. As I observed earlier, after 1970, labor markets and the labor process became restructured while the technology used in production became more adaptable; mass production and standardized products gave way to custom marketing, directed toward a variety of niches (Smith 1991). Firms that made use of new microelectronic technologies, integrating design, production, marketing, and distribution, "could produce small quantities of high-quality, semi-customized goods

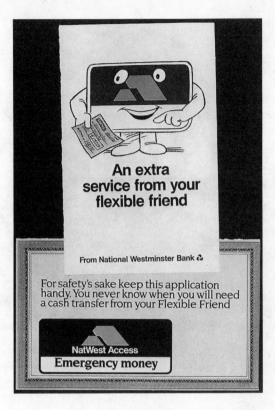

Fig. 23. *A NatWest credit card, "your flexible friend." (Thanks to Marilyn Strathern for giving me this brochure.)*

Fig. 24. *Chase Manhattan's flexible credit card. Their credit plan allows the consumer flexible choice, lowering or raising credit limits, skipping up to two payments a year. (Still from a television ad provided thanks to the help of Aubrey E. Hawes, vice president, Chase Manhattan Bank. Thanks to Mary Poovey for telling me about the Chase ad campaign centered around the concept of flexibility.)*

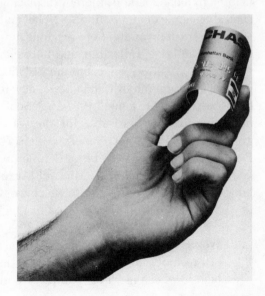

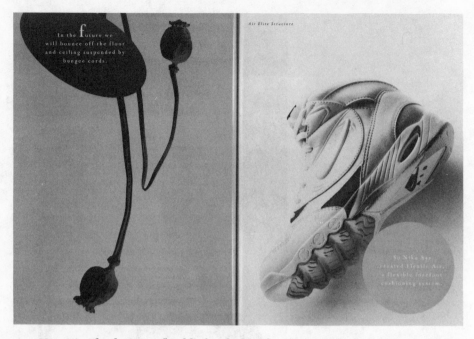

Fig. 25. *Flexile Air, a flexible forefoot cushioning system from Nike shoes, useful for bouncing off the floor and ceiling suspended by bungee cords. From* Shape, *February 1993, following p.32.*

tailored to niche markets, thereby displacing economies of scale as the central dynamic of competition" (Nolan and O'Donnell 1991:161).

These small firms are more dynamic, innovative, and responsive to change than large, inflexible, and bureaucratic conglomerates; they require a committed, educated, multiskilled workforce, able to learn new abilities continuously and take up new functions as the market dictates (Nolan and O'Donnell 1991:162). Sentiment about whether these developments are desirable for the well-being of workers varies greatly, from Piore and Sabel's (1984:17–18) early enthusiasm to Pollert's (1991:161) recent bitter skepticism.

New Age Philosophy. In Michael Murphy's encyclopedic source book *The Future of the Body*, to which we will turn again later, bodily flexibility is a sign of having evolved to a higher order of being:

> We can extrapolate from physiological changes revealed by modern research in imagining somatic developments required for high-level change. For example, we might guess that molecular

and atomic interactions within cells are altered to facilitate extraordinary vitality and movement. The marvelous flexibility exhibited by sports-people in certain inspired performances, the astonishing distortions of limbs and torso experienced by some Catholic saints and the breathtaking agility of certain dancers and shamans indicate that muscles, tendons, and ligaments are, under some conditions, capable of extraordinary elasticity. Might such elasticity be taken to new levels still? (Murphy 1992:157)

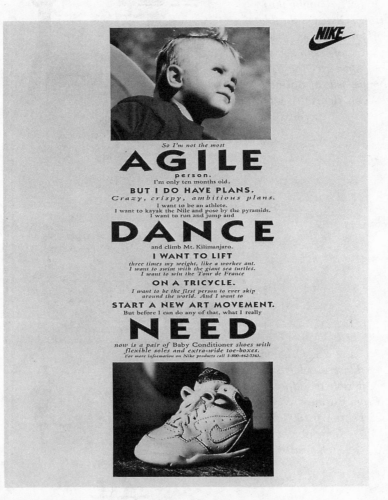

Fig. 26. *Baby Conditioner with flexible soles from Nike. From* Parenting, *May 1992, inside back cover. Reprinted with permission of Nike, Inc. (Photo by Enrique Badalescu.)*

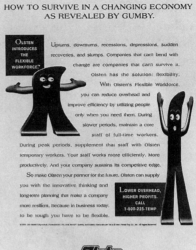

Fig. 27. *Gumby illustrates Olsten's "flexible workforce." From p. 209 of "Reinventing America," the 1992 bonus issue of* Business Week. *Reprinted with permission.*

Fig. 28. *Origami illustrates Olsten's "flexible workforce." From* Business Week, *22 February 1993, 22. Reprinted with permission.*

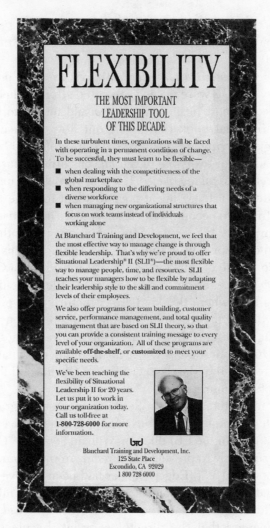

Fig. 29. *Flexibility makes the headline in an ad for a training and development firm. From* Training and Development, *April 1992, 8.*

The desire for bodily flexibility over strength alone is also expressed in many other publications more oriented toward a mass audience. The *Amtrak Express* reports that, while the 1970s was the decade of aerobics and the 1980s the decade of weight training, the 1990s will be the decade of stretching (Walters 1993:18). The article quotes a tai chi master on the benefits of stretching: "So much of the goal [in Western culture] is to be stronger or faster or more powerful, instead of more fluid, more resilient, more healthy, more organic." With stretching for flexibility, our movements can become "a dance in its most organic form" (p. 19).

Government Organizations. In Baltimore over the period of my research, city officials were making concerted efforts to help city organizations become more flexible, innovative, and anticipatory. I was told that one influential book that spells out how this can be done, *Reinventing Government* (Osborne and Gaebler 1992), became required reading for everyone in the mayor's office. This book summarizes the changes taking place: "It is as if virtually all institutions in American life were struggling at once to adapt to some massive sea change — striving to become more flexible, more innovative, and more entrepreneurial" (p. 12). Consultants and visitors from other city governments and major corporations in the United States (including Rockford Co., a site of my fieldwork that I introduce in Chapter 11) came to give advice, as did representatives of local councils in the United Kingdom, where this kind of restructuring is well advanced. Toward the end of my research, complex linkages to encourage the restructuring of organizations were being built among the mayor's office, the Human Resources Department of my university, corporations in the region, the Maryland Center for Quality and Productivity, and the Clinton administration.

Just how much the "virtue" of flexibility is taken for granted in the way in which government functions is shown in the media response to Clinton's dismissal of the FBI director, William Sessions: "Congress set a 10-year term partly to prevent the director from becoming as independently powerful as J. Edgar Hoover had been for five decades; it expected that leadership changes would occur in the mid-terms of administrations rather than the outset. Still, for *vital flexibility*, Congress decreed that the director serve at the pleasure of the President" ("Change at the Top" 1993:A4). Or again, Senator Daniel Patrick Moynihan made it into boldface type on the front page of the *New York Times* because, in insisting that Clinton compromise during negotiations over the administration's budget plan, Moynihan was "pushing for flexibility." In the article within, the reporter implies that Moynihan's dire accusation of "inflexibility" had an immediate effect. By the end of the day, Moynihan said, the administration was demonstrating much more willingness to collaborate (Rosenbaum 1993).

Psychology. In the 1980s and 1990s, two academic psychologists, whose work has been widely received, began to publish about the flexible, ever-shifting self, which some of us are lucky enough to have.[8] For Mihaly Csikszentmihalyi, some people, born with a "more focussed and flexible neurological endowment," are able to achieve an "autotelic" self, a self in which the goals that one pursues arise from within: "On the one hand, having a feeling of ownership of her decisions, the person is more strongly dedicated to her goals. Her actions are reliable and internally controlled. On the other hand, knowing them to be her own, she can more easily modify her goals whenever the reasons for preserving them no longer make sense. In that respect, an autotelic person's behavior is both more consistent and more flexible" (Csikszentmihalyi 1990:209–10).

For Kenneth Gergen, a self is emerging whose "persistent identity cannot seem to be fixed": "One swims in ever-shifting, concatenating, and contentious currents of being" (1991:80). Gergen's work has been used in the popular press to assert that: "Americans no longer look to men of steel — we want honest and flexible leaders" (Anderson 1993:95).[9]

New definitions of human intelligence also began to emerge from social psychology, stressing its flexibly adaptive character: "It is purposive, flexibly attuned to the goals most salient in each problem context, not rigidly stereotyped or indiscriminate in nature" (Cantor and Kihlstrom 1987:47). "Social intelligence" is a type of intelligence that demands a high degree of flexibility. The first issue of the new journal *Social Intelligence* explains that the journal will be "a vehicle to explore techniques, technology platforms and training tactics which allow social operators to see things differently, with multiple vision. The emphasis is on flexibility and faceting" (quoted in Strathern, in press).

Feminism. Sonia Johnson, feminist and excommunicated Mormon, argues that women can change the system. How? "In order to survive at all, women have had to become almost preternaturally flexible. Our outsider status also gives us flexibility. Being by definition outside the system, no matter how inside it we may wish or perceive ourselves to be, and having no genuine stake in it, gives us very real freedoms of intellect and spirit. The oppressed, always most outside the system and always most flexible, are therefore always the controlling elements in any system" (Johnson 1987:319). Johnson is attempting to use flexibility subversively. She is imagining the unforeseen ways in which a person unconstrained by being within a system can move and act and therefore how this flexibility could enable someone to influence the system from outside.

Chela Sandoval, a feminist theorist, argues for an "oppositional consciousness" informed by the theoretical perspectives of Third World feminists:

> Its power can be thought of as mobile — not nomadic but rather cinematographic: a kinetic motion that maneuvers, poetically transfigures, and orchestrates while demanding alienation, perversion, and reformation in both spectators and practitioners. . . . Differential consciousness requires grace, flexibility, and strength: enough strength to confidently commit to a well-defined structure of identity for one hour, day, week, month, year; enough flexibility to self-consciously transform that identity according to the requisites of another oppositional ideological tactic if readings of power's formation require it, enough grace to recognize alliance with others committed to egalitarian social relations and race, gender, and class justice when their readings of power call for alternative oppositional stands. (Sandoval 1991:3, 15)

Sandoval is extolling the active, initiating, mobile aspects of flexibility. Not surprisingly, these two feminists, of very different persuasions, are equally enamored of the quality of flexibility, given its many valences. Depending on whether one is gaining flexibility as a necessity of surviving while being powerless or as an adjunct of developing new, less repressive forms of interaction, flexibility seems to be the key. These are the opposed extremes of the social positions in which women so commonly find themselves, on the one hand, and wish they could be more often, on the other.

Observing ethnographically the seductiveness of flexibility as a quality in a great many domains, I turned back to a book I had not read for many years, Gregory Bateson's *Steps to an Ecology of Mind* (1972), which was written at the beginning of the period of flexible specialization. Since I was (finally) beginning to grasp the importance of the preeminence given to the quality of flexibility in the 1990s, as our culture has come to think of the world and the self in terms of complex systems, I was captivated by Bateson's much earlier account of how complex systems are organized. His account ends with the chapter "Ecology and Flexibility in Urban Civilization." Bateson asserts, "To achieve, in a few generations, anything like the healthy system dreamed of above or even to get out of the grooves of fatal destiny in which our civilization is now caught, very great *flexibility* will be needed. It is right, therefore, to examine this concept with some care. Indeed, this is a crucial concept" (p. 496). Bateson goes on to compare a healthy system to "an acrobat on a high wire": "To maintain the ongoing truth of his basic premise ('I am on the wire'), he must be free to move from one position of instability to another, i.e., certain variables such as the position of his arms and the rate of movement of his arms must have great flexibility, which he uses to maintain the stability of other more fundamental and general characteristics" (p. 498).

With great prescience, Bateson aptly captured the notion of the flexible, constantly adjusting, constantly changing person, long before its appearance in ads for athletic shoes and temporary employment services. In subsequent chapters, we will see how flexibility comes to play a role in our cultural ideas about who will be able to survive into the future at all.

PART
FIVE

PRACTICUMS

PRACTICUM: N. Amer. A practical exercise; a course of practical training.

The Oxford English Dictionary

IF SCIENTIFIC KNOWLEDGE IS TO HAVE AN EFFECT BEYOND THE LAB-oratory, it must enter other contexts, instantiated in the form of writing, action, regulations, or institutions. If scientists' discoveries in the lab are to have a chance to affect other scientists, they must, among other things, write, talk, publish, lecture, and teach about them. If scientific findings are to be taken up by nonscientists in the wider society, then it helps if, among other things, reporters write about them, artists draw pictures of them, photographers photograph them, states enforce the use of them, inventors build them into their products, and schools teach about them. In this part, we will examine several practices that are important in mediating the relations between cultural understand-ings in the wider society and scientific research on the immune system.

Bruno Latour has discussed how written inscriptions help form and solidify scientific knowledge in scientific communities. They become more powerful the more they are printed, two dimensional, flat, immutable, and recombinable (Latour 1986:20). In laboratories, initial messy data are organized into patterns, simplified, and eventually visu-ally represented in a table or graph. Although Latour argues convinc-ingly that these graphic tracings are what have the most powerful effects in science, I am less convinced by his claim that the model can be extended to all of society: "What is this society in which a written, printed mathematical form has greater credence, in case of doubt, than anything else: common sense, the senses other than vision, political authority, tradition, and even the Scriptures?" (p. 26).

In my research "in this society" for this book, I've found that the printed mathematical form is not preeminent outside the specialized world of the laboratory and the scientist. We have already seen material in previous chapters demonstrating that the static, two-dimensional, flat model of the health of the body is not what is being given currency in the popular imagination. Configurations involving flexible, complex systems are in fact diametrically opposed to flat, static models. They are by definition in constant motion, continually changing, and multidimensional: hence it is a challenge to represent these models in the print media. Vera Michaels, who drew "the wave" to represent the immune system, evokes with graphic simplicity the complexity and turbulence of the action of waves. The power of her drawing is not in its reduced, immutable form but in its suggestiveness; it points to something that is the opposite of immutability. In contrast, laboratory inscriptions work in a very different way: they point away from the complex messiness of the experimental work that preceded them toward a simple, immutable form.[1]

Laboratory inscriptions rely completely on the primacy of vision. This is not surprising because, in Western culture, vision has long been the sense given a privileged position by the exploring scientist, for whom results must be seen and replicated to be properly understood. As will become clear in the next chapter, my research reconfirms yet again the primacy of the link between knowledge and "seeing." But dealing with complex systems involves more than reducing them to flat, static graphs or formulas. Scientists and mathematicians, to be sure, may continue to wrestle the nature of complex systems into the strictures of mathematical formulas, but increasingly they are becoming engaged — and engage us — with the mystery of a form that is always the same and always different: the fractal. The issue of *Immunology Today* that promoted the possibility that the immune system may be a complex system had a color image of a fractal on its cover. The many popular science books on complex systems almost inevitably include color plates of fractals, images that seem to catch an ever-changing kaleidoscope in motion (Gleick 1987).

In this part, we will see how people who are not scientists engage these configurations in a number of ways. Visual materials play an important role, to be sure. But alongside them we will find rich varieties of multisensory experiences. Alongside *seeing* will be *hearing*, *smelling*, *feeling*, *tasting*, and an enormous range of emotional states, from fear and sadness, to despair and joy. As we saw in the powerful effect of the HIV– but AIDS+ patients, whose sick bodies and failed immune systems disrupted the steady march of science at the Eighth International AIDS Conference in Amsterdam, flat and static graphs are not the only entities that wield power.

Interestingly, one kind of image that is very frequently used to convey scientific findings both among scientists and between scientists and the public is the electron micrograph. This is a *photograph* that captures a three-dimensional form in one plane. As we will see, these photographs are understood by many people in poetic, emotional, multisensory ways.

CHAPTER 8

Interpreting Electron Micrographs

I think I felt as I would if a doctor had held an X-ray to the light showing a star-shaped hole at the center of one of my vital organs. Death has entered. It is inside you. You are said to be dying and yet are separate from the dying, can ponder it at your leisure, literally see on the X-ray photograph or computer screen the horrible alien logic of it all. It is when death is rendered graphically, is televised so to speak, that you sense an eerie separation between your condition and yourself. A network of symbols has been introduced, an entire awesome technology wrested from the gods. It makes you feel like a stranger in your own dying.

DON DELILLO, *White Noise*

When I was doing the research for this book, I frequently attended lectures on immunology in classrooms and lecture halls. Almost inevitably, the lecturer would illustrate his or her statements with slides and transparencies depicting a microscopic view of the cell or process being described. Various tiny participants in the immune system (T cells, antibodies, tissue stricken by autoimmune reactions) would suddenly loom huge on the screen in the lecture room, dwarfing us all. Often the rhetorical flow of the lecture was timed to produce these images at a moment of closure and proof: this is what I say we found, and *here is a picture of it!* In one striking case, where the lecturer was able to illustrate a process that he had discovered experimentally with a videotape of the cells actually engaged in the process, the audience audibly gasped in appreciation.[1]

There is certainly a lively aesthetic involved when scientists produce, choose, and display these images. After many a lecture, I heard people commenting to each other about the "beautiful," "incredible," "stunning," "technically perfect" micrographs that were shown. The standards of the scientific community are so high, researchers told me, that (for fear of ridicule) one would never dare use an image that was imperfect: one that showed extraneous dirt, one that was blurry, one that showed any degradation from the tissue-fixing process. But aside from this (a topic about which a great deal more could be said!), the main thrust of the pictures in science is to clinch an argument by revealing visual evidence of what one is claiming.[2] In the immunology lab where I did fieldwork, this was impressed on me in many ways. One researcher lamented that the photographs accompanying his articles could not be as convincing as those of his colleagues who used micrographs of cells: as I have mentioned, his findings depended on the Western blot, a technique that he was teaching me, and, however well it was done, it could result only in fuzzy and indistinct bands in vague shades of gray. Another researcher recalled the turning point in immunology when Gerald Edelman, a Nobel Prize recipient, saw for the first time a micrograph of an antibody, which forced him to revise his own calculations about antibody structure. Photographs, especially electron micrographs, are used to achieve closure and finality in scientific arguments.[3]

Outside research science, I noticed that electron micrographs illustrating biological processes appear in a great variety of popular publications.[4] Whole books are devoted to revealing the invisible world of microbes and microorganisms that live among us: for example, *Microcosmos* (Burgess, Marten, and Taylor 1987) and *The Secret House* (Bodanis 1986). Ordinary household appliances have been redesigned specifically to rid our homes of these unwanted guests; advertisements for vacuum cleaners with special filters are now commonly accompanied by electron micrographs of the dust mite, which is a common cause of allergies. Films and textbooks on biology for schools covering topics from asthma to reproduction frequently include many micrographs illustrating cells, viruses, etc. and their activities.[5]

Electron microscopy played a starring role in a popular article about a potentially disastrous outbreak of an infectious virus brought into the

United States by way of African monkeys intended for scientific research. Electron micrographs of cells from one of the monkeys' livers provide "definite confirmation" that the cells are infected with a filovirus, a type of virus that includes Ebola virus, known to have been lethal to almost nine of ten humans who contracted it in previous outbreaks in Africa (Preston 1992:71). In the end, the filovirus in the United States turned out to be a variant of the deadly Ebola that was not harmful to humans. But the four Hollywood movie studios who wanted to offer Richard Preston, the author of the article, a contract for the film rights to the story apparently intended to make the electron microscope as sleuth a central feature of the plot.[6] (We will have to wait and see whether 20th Century Fox, which won the contract, follows through.)

As I became aware of the extent to which electron micrographs have pervaded our popular culture, I decided to include a series of interactions with electron micrographs in the general interviews on health that we were conducting in urban neighborhoods. When a conversation with someone was off to a good start, we would show him or her a series of micrographs of cells involving the immune system (see fig. 30*a*–*b*). We would say that these were enlarged photographs of things inside the body and ask in one way or another, "What do you make of this?" If the person hesitated to say anything, wanting more specific information from us, the interviewer would read aloud the brief caption that appeared with the photograph in the original publication.[7]

One of our goals was to see how familiar people were with these images perambulating out from science into the society, in what Bruno Latour calls the "irruption of objects into the human collective" (1990:152). Another goal was to see whether, even though the images were usually taken to have been produced by and within the rational world of science and scientists, people would dare speak about them imaginatively. Often we would ask, "Do these pictures bring any thoughts to mind?" or, "How do you react to these pictures?" We were interested in whether people would have anything to say at all, given the strong authority with which science speaks in our culture, and given the strong antithesis between the taken-for-granted rationality and certainty of scientific knowledge and what we were asking for: imaginatively produced interpretations.

In due course, we would also ask whether having seen the images we introduced or other similar ones might change the way in which the

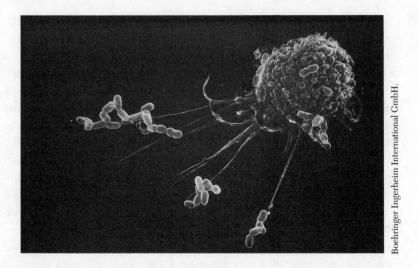

Fig. 30. *Electron micrographs of immune system cells. a, Mutiny in the body: T cells surrounding a tumor cell. b, First step in phagocytosis. From P. Jaret, "The Wars Within,"* National Geographic, *June 1986, 725 and 718 respectively.*

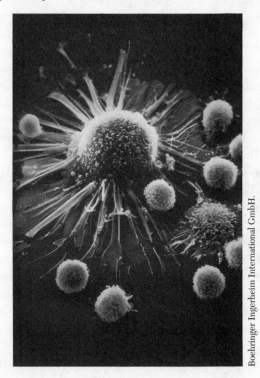

person thought about his or her body or self. Obviously, asking such questions so bluntly and in such a confined context has limited utility. The results presented below should be taken as only an initial indication of the kind of impact that these images may be having in our society generally.

Much attention has been paid in social studies of science to ways in which scientific machines and their operations and tests can become "obligatory passage points" for the conduct of science (Latour 1983, 1987). In an example that Latour interprets as a case of a scientific invention becoming an obligatory passage point, in the seventeenth century Robert Boyle was able to make witnesses' observations of his air pump a necessary adjudicator of diverse questions: "Discussions about the Body Politic, God and His miracles, Matter and its power, could be *made to go* through the air pump" (Latour 1990:152; see also Shapin and Schaffer 1985). Scientists, theologians, and philosophers came to treat the results of observation of the air pump as decisive in their discussions: submitting their questions to the facts that the air pump could reveal became obligatory.[8]

Latour often argues that the force of these scientific tools that become obligatory passage points resides in their ability to effect a change in scale: "the essential feature of modern power: change of scale and displacement through workshop and laboratories" (Latour 1990:153). In the change of scale, something *very minute*, discovered by science, comes to play a deciding role in human questions or concerns that are *very large*.

For the most part, in our research we found that micrographs were what might be called *weakly obligatory* passage points. Their ubiquity meant that most people had bumped into them before. But, in one context of our fieldwork, contact with images and knowledge about cellular entities were *strongly obligatory*: a college class on cancer and AIDS taught by a molecular biologist in a large state university. A member of our ethnographic research group took the course and interviewed the professor and a selection of the students.[9] I begin with a discussion of this context because, unlike the people in our general interviews, the students in this class were literally being tested on how well they absorbed the professor's view of what makes up the body.

The professor, whom I will call Peter Keller, had a clear message that he wanted to convey to students:

I think one's attitude toward one's health is enormously important to determining one's health. So without really trying, just by
studying the immune system . . . you have this stuff. Your B lymphocytes are incredible. I think they're saying, "Oh!" and you
almost stand up a little taller, and you walk around and say, "I'm
powerful," which I think is extremely useful in being powerful
and being healthy. So I just in some sense consciously identify
with powerful things in me. . . . If you got a group of twenty people together and said, "You know what you have in you? You have
this immune system. You know what it can do? I mean you know
why a vaccine works? You know why you only get a cold, a disease only once?" And, "Wow, really? I have that in me?" It seems
to me, I just take that for very granted that that is empowering
and makes people stronger.

But, in spite of his strong agenda and his role as teacher, the students had a wide range of different responses to images of cells of the
immune system. One student echoes the professor's message: "I don't
think the average person realizes, you know, what your body does. I
mean, it's such a gigantic task to take care of these things, All this stuff's
going on, so much all the time. I think we just take a lot for granted,
but it really is kind of neat" (Drew Stratton). Another reflects back on
how much he was influenced by the class when he took it two years ago
but rejects altogether the link that Professor Keller takes for granted
between the biological details and feeling empowered:

With all the lingo that was going on, the technical, the different
types of cells, all the interaction within the system, I don't know
if that just turned me off or —
The technical language?
Yeah. . . . I just lost interest, or I thought of it as something
physical, and I didn't really see any connection. . . . It just
seemed like too much was known, or not that a lot was known,
but maybe since I couldn't relate to that, I felt that that couldn't
help me, so I didn't take anything from it. I mean, just all the
names and all the different processes involved. I didn't really
care about it.
Really, that's interesting.
Just maybe it's because if someone comes and names all the different processes and explains how they work, but as far as using

that for my own good, or. . . . And I think that's one of the reasons why I got a C. (Laughs.) It's true. I barely got a C at that.
. . . I got a lot out of the course, but just not as far as the technical lingo and all the different processes involved. (Mike
Franzini)

Other students acknowledged the impact of knowledge about the
cells of the immune system but felt that it *reduced* their sense of
empowerment and control. Recall Martha Novick, whom we met in
Chapter 5, saying:

I could think, like, I have more control because, you know, there
are things you can do to affect something that's going on in your
body, but then you think you could be in less control because
there's so many other things in your body that, maybe, you don't
know about. And they just go on constantly without even you
thinking about them. So that I guess that could make you think
that I was, like, in less control, too. A whole other world.

Others, too, find it difficult to feel that the enlarged images are really
part of them, much less that they are empowered by knowledge about
them:

It's actually hard for me to picture these things in my body. I
mean I'm sure they're there, but, you know, seeing them so, so
big, I mean this is really scary. And, I mean, this up close is. . . .
I mean they're so microscopic, you know what I mean? That
when you magnify it by a certain amount, it's scary. But I mean
I can't really associate these things inside my body. It's kind of
hard for me to. Like when the pictures go away, I won't really,
you know, I'll see them, but I won't really still —
You won't identify with them?
Not really. (Cary Lennox)

This brief introduction suggests the wide latitude of reactions to
electron micrographs, even in circumstances where an authority figure
is suggesting a particular interpretation. Given this, we thought that
the people we interviewed in the neighborhoods would offer many different interpretations of micrographs. But their responses exceeded
our expectations extravagantly. Taken as a whole, the things that people

said can be described only as a profusion, an excess of images.
Sometimes they tumble out one close on top of another:

> Sort of like a landscape, perhaps coralish, maybe a seascape or
> something. . . . Sort of a crystal quality. . . . The cancer cell looks
> sort of like a puff pastry, doesn't it, and this looks like a Dunkin'
> Donut hole with coconut on it. (Bill Slocum)

> Those remind me like a plant, it looks like a plant. These look like
> somebody being at sea, you know what I'm saying? Like they call
> those jellyfish and stuff like that — plants that be in the sea.
> (Tyrone Walter)

> This looks like something's shooting out of it, trying to kill
> the other one, kind of almost *Star Wars*–ish . . . almost like a
> frog or a toad or whatever; it has a long tongue that shoots out
> and gets flies. . . . Sputnik! a satellite would be the other thing
> that it conjures up . . . or something undersea, Jacques Cousteau–
> ish. . . . Something like an alien. . . . I like this one better because
> it takes it inside. It's a little more like some sort of knight being
> the champion and engulfing it and killing it as opposed to the
> other one being almost like a leech and attaching itself and then
> killing it, killing it, more like a tick, I don't like ticks of course.
> (Charles Kingsley)

Sometimes specific photographs elicited extended commentary. For
example, we showed Tara Holcolm a picture of how arthritis affects the
bone and asked:

> *Could you explain to me again what you think is happening*
> *with the arthritis?*
> It looked like a desert that collects sand through here and then
> this rock, and this right here kind of like a little eye and a ear,
> like an animal that's fighting for its life. Or maybe like a little
> baby animal, the eye and the nose right here, that can't do too
> much for himself, or like fossils of what used to be. A monster
> through here. This looks like wasted land, maybe something
> after maybe a bomb hits.

When we showed Sally Felton a picture of a white blood cell and a tumor cell, she responded:

> Yeah, you can look at a picture like this and just get a feeling for almost the psychology of these things, tumor cells just like gobbling up nutrients and taking over from healthy tissue. I mean this reflects a sort of malevolence that, I don't know, I just think of tumors in that way, and you know, this poor little white cell here, it's like, the sucker doesn't stand a chance.
> *This is bacteria, and, let me see, this is the explanation;* this *is* this *enlarged.*
> It's almost evocative of like patriarchal notions of conquest. This is like the United States invading Panama, right here. Except in this case, the little suckers really do need to be kept in check.

Showing him a picture of a white blood cell and bacteria, we asked Horace Miner:

> *So what do they make you feel or think of? What do they remind you of?*
> I guess that's what cells would look like inside your body. Looks like it's trying to do something, get away from something, or something. . . . They look like spiders trying to catch flies on a web or something.
> *A spider? Oh, yeah.*
> Trying to catch an ant or something . . . This one looks like it's getting bigger or whatever. . . . So does this one.
> *What?*
> I say it's trying to grow.

It was very evident throughout our interviews that many people do not hesitate to exercise their imaginations when confronted by the photographic tracings of scientific knowledge. This is so in spite of the awe that many people expressed at this knowledge and the scientists who produced it. Many people commented on the amazing powers of scientists who have the ability to make pictures like these: "It makes me marvel at what we are, not only . . . that this exists inside our bodies, but that we as humans have been able to photograph these. I think that's kind of neat" (George Miller).

When we look in more detail at the reflections inspired by micrographs, we see clearly the potential of the micrographs to mobilize a great variety of emotional and conceptual positions. They encourage *empathy* with the pain of the illnesses that they depict:

> ***Do you think when you look at pictures like this, do you think that's changed at all how you see your body?***
> I think so. First of all the pictures of the arthritis make my understanding of that and of what Linda's fighting off a lot more graphic. It makes that more real, what arthritis is, and gives me a better sense of understanding the kind of pain that she can have with it . . . seeing that. It looks painful. (Cindy Radlaw)

They elicit *awe* at the processes going on within the body:

> ***When you see these kind of photos, I mean at the really micro, micro level, and you think about them in terms like this, does it change the way you think about your body?***
> Yeah. I think you forget what's really going on in there. What really you're made up of, it's awesome. I mean it's fascinating to me. It's awesome. It makes me realize how incredible the human body is, you know, what's really going on in there. You walk around every day, you exist, but what's really happening to you? (Elizabeth Houlihan)

They inspire *appreciation* of how actively the body is always working:

> ***Does it make you think differently about your own body when you see pictures like that?***
> Like this picture, what it makes me feel like is that my body is very active, in what it can do. And, because I feel my body functioning at times, I feel like, yeah, we're doing all right. If I have a bruise, if I've bumped myself or something, and I see a bruise, and then the next day I notice that it's faded, that does make me feel good about my body because I feel as though things are working.
> ***So you can sort of imagine these things going on?***
> Going *zap!* Space invaders. (Lisa Demarco)

You think about the body as being, if you think about it, and you don't do it that often, unless it's acting up, and you really don't think about it, you just take for granted that all these things are working, the heart is pumping and the blood's flowing. You take it for granted, till something goes wrong. But to think that there is so much activity, it's like a city, like a little city, you know? (Judy Lockard)

In the midst of so much appreciative evaluation of micrographs and their effects, many people could also see another, and more ambiguous, effect of these images. Sometimes the lability of the images, the very fact that like ink blots they could represent anything at all, overwhelms the instructions with which they come — that they depict what is really happening inside us. Some people almost refuse to believe that they are pictures of the body's interior:

> *When you see these kind of photos, does it change the way that you think about your body?*
> . . . Seeing it, at this magnification, it takes on almost a surreal look to it so that it doesn't seem quite real. So much so that, even though it exists, it looks like something otherworldly. . . . A photograph of this nature doesn't have as much effect as seeing someone with a full-blown case of AIDS or something like that. Show a before-and-after picture. But make sure that the before is a happy picture. . . . These, you know, there's nothing that anyone could look at and say, "Yeah, I've seen that before," or, "That's me." (George Miller)

To George Miller, the micrograph is too foreign and alien. In his view, a representation of the body of a person with a full-blown case of AIDS would connect with him more powerfully than a "surreal," "otherworldly" micrograph of HIV.

Phillip Monroe was probably the most verbally enthusiastic when looking at the micrographs. Over and over again he said that they were "phenomenal," "fascinating," "incredible." Even so, he also experienced a surreal sense of disconnection to the processes that they illustrated:

It's like being in two different worlds.
Really?
Yeah, I mean, even though I've seen all these kinds of things
before and I realize that these are the exact same kinds of
things that are in my body, it's still distanced somehow, and I
think it's because . . . these cells act on their own, you know.
There's no connection between . . . me being a conscious
human being and this cell that's inside me.

For Phillip Monroe, the cells are very small in scale, and their importance to "a conscious human being" is also very small. This reaction
seems to work in the opposite direction to Bruno Latour's notions
about how science sometimes works by modifying the relative scale of
phenomena. As Latour explains, changing the relative scale of phenomena means, in the case of Boyle's air pump, making something that
scientists have discovered that is very small in scale come to have a very
large, decisive role in the world:

> Boyle modifies the *relative scale* of phenomena: macro-factors
> about matter and God's powers may be made amenable to an
> experimental solution and this solution will be a partial modest
> one. . . . [Boyle] refines his experiment to show the effect on a
> detector — a feather! — of the aether wind postulated by
> Hobbes thus hoping to disprove his contradictor. How ridiculous!
> Hobbes raises a big problem and he is rebutted by a feather
> inside a transparent glass inside a laboratory inside Boyle's man-
> sion! (Latour 1990:153)

But Phillip Monroe refuses to accept the reversal of scale, which would
subordinate him as a conscious human being to the tiny cells within.
For other people, the scale reversal is so fascinating that they carry it
one step further and imagine that we humans might be "cells" inside
something very large:

> Maybe we're a part of something so big that it doesn't know that
> we exist. You know, and we're just going along, just like these cells
> are going along. . . . And so, you know, it's just like maybe these
> cells don't even know that they're a part of a body, which is weird,
> but maybe they don't, you know? Maybe they're just doing this
> function because it's what's programmed into them, but they

don't know, you know, Oh, I'm part of Bob or, you know, whatever. They don't know this. So like that we don't know that we're part of something bigger. We're just going along doing what we believe to be what we're supposed to do or whatever. (Brackette Thompson)

Whether the scale reversal is relished or rejected, the ability of the images to create and sustain a sense of distance from one's own body is palpable. The theme of distance is shot through many of the comments above: the images involve "separation," one "can't relate" to them, they are "like a whole other world," it is "hard to picture" these things in one's body, they are "distanced," they and we are in "two different worlds," they are "surreal, otherworldly."

As DEPICTIONS of the body, micrographs show microscopic entities radically decontextualized from the context of the body. In speaking of the creation of distance between the colonial British and the inhabitants of India, Bernard Cohn refers to the role of *depiction* in establishing and maintaining a power differential: "Indians [are depicted] as isolated, *decontextualized objects* whose meaning can only be inferred from their special dress or the presence of the tools of their trades, and displaying the markers of the services which they were to provide to the sahibs and memsabibs" (quoted in Corrigan 1988:267). The depiction removes Indians from their culture and marks them with the trappings of —"tethers them" to — colonialism. Similarly, the micrograph depicts decontextualized parts of the body and marks them with the trappings of — "tethers them" to — science. What our interviews show is that the *decontextualization* "takes" more often than the tethering to science. The depictions in micrographs are so decontextualized that they could be anything at all, from jellyfish in the ocean deep, to star wars in outer space.

Up to this point, I have treated the neighborhood interviews as a kind of collective text produced by nonscientists. Although there were obviously a great many kinds of interpretations, there was no grouping based on gender, age, ethnicity, class, or residence in the nearly two hundred interviews that did not show engagement with the micrographs in the intense ways I described above. We also found similarly intense involvement among those we interviewed who were political activists, AIDS/HIV activists, and community leaders. There was, however, one exceptional case in which a man rejected the micrographs roundly, finding them irrelevant to his and his community's life. John Marcellino is a community leader in Warren, a neighborhood with high unemployment and pervasive poverty: he runs a center that provides the community with resources, including educational classes and social service referrals. When John first saw the photographs, he said, "That's disgusting. . . . [Laughs.] That's very mystical. . . . I mean I know that's really amazing. It's like looking up into the sky at night, you know what I mean, and really thinking about it. I mean, I know that's really amazing. . . . You don't learn about this kind of stuff, you know, in school or anything like that. They don't teach you about this kind of stuff, so I don't understand it. But I know it's pretty amazing." But, in spite of his amazement, John goes on to emphasize the distance that separates him and his community from the scientists who have produced these images:

> See, we don't talk to many scientists . . . you know, so I don't get to hear that much stuff. This is not a conversation that includes us. I tell you that most of our people don't.
> *No.*
> You show these pictures, somebody's going to think that it's some spaced-out artist, you know what I mean? People have no idea what this conversation is about. You know what I'm saying?
> *Yeah, but you watched a National Geographic [film called* The Miracle of Life]?
> Yeah.
> *So what I was wondering is that, after watching that, or after seeing pictures like this, does that change in any way the way you think about your body or about yourself?*
> For a little while, probably. But not permanent I don't think.
> *In what way would it be very little?*
> Because it's too much to comprehend, I guess, because I didn't get enough information to really understand it. Though I understood it more than when we started talking. [Laughs.] But I mean, probably because I don't really understand it, I understand it in different terms, you know.

Faced with the social realities of the poverty and ill health that are pervasive in Warren, John finds the esoteric knowledge of the interior of the body irrelevant: "It's really interesting, but it's not important at all":

> I've had people die of cancer, I guess I'm still more concerned with how they feel, and their part in life, and how they're going to go into death, than I am about what is going on with this disease inside of your body or their body. You know? I don't know if that makes sense, but how this thing works is kind of, it's really interesting, but it's not, it's not important at all. You know what I mean?
> **Yeah, I know what you mean.**
> I mean, what's important is all this stuff out here we're trying to deal with. And if I didn't have anything else to do, I mean I could just watch videos about it for a long time, you know. I would love to talk to people about it. I'd like to learn more.

Biological science relentlessly pushes the level of its analysis down to a scale below the level of human lived experience, to the microscopic level of microbes, cells, or genes. Marcellino is able both to feel the attraction and force of knowledge about events happening at that level ("It's interesting. . . . I'd like to know more") and to articulate the irrelevance of the microscopic level to the reality of human lives. To do this he has constantly to pull the level of discussion up from the microscopic scale to the human scale. For the people in his community who "have no idea what this conversation is about," he is "more concerned with . . . their part in life, and how they're going to go into death," than with what is going on with the cells inside their bodies.

We talked to many others who were politically active in their communities, but no one else articulated a connection between attention paid to microscopic cells and a lack of attention to social problems. Marcellino's singular observations surely speak to his own acuity as well as to the mesmerizing effect of micrographs imbued with the power of scientific knowledge.

The predicament affecting John Marcellino, even with his particularly adroit ability to confront the knowledge produced by science, is that the most energetic effort to "pull" the scale of knowledge up above the microscopic still cannot cancel out the impact of having seen things at the microscopic level. Once the body has been seen that way, our interviews suggest, the experience is not easily forgotten. The experience is also frequently reevoked, as we will see, by the "saturation" of the visual field in media and teaching materials with micrographs and by processes like testing (whether a college examination or a T cell count) that increasingly make knowledge of the microscopic biological entities inside us something inescapable.

These encounters with micrographs show us that the scientific questions impelling production of these images are not necessarily the questions that grip nonscientific people as they marvel at them, reject their relevance, or integrate them creatively into ordinary life. Micrographs are used to produce closure in arguments among scientists; when people outside science respond to them, they result in anything *but* closure. Instead, there is a kind of efflorescence of variation: what for one person is a dreadful prospect — like DeLillo's "horrible alien logic," "an entire awesome technology wrested from the gods" that makes you "a stranger in your own dying" — is, for another, a spectacle filled with awe and, for another, simply a mildly interesting byproduct of a scientific conversation that ignores what is most important: the social and economic conditions that lead to suffering and illness in a poor urban neighborhood.

CHAPTER 9

Saturation

> *In our Anglo-American society — a relatively indoor one — when a performance is given it is usually given in a highly bounded region, to which boundaries with respect to time are often added. The impression and understanding fostered by the performance will tend to saturate the region and time span, so that any individual located in this space-time manifold will be in a position to observe the performance and be guided by the definition of the situation which the performance fosters.*
>
> ERVING GOFFMAN, *The Presentation of Self in Everyday Life*

In this chapter, I continue to explore the ways in which a certain picture of the body as a complex system comes to have powerful effects on our lives. Recalling what we learned about complex systems in Chapter 5, I argue that the immune system has come to be a kind of "field" of health, in Hayles's sense that "reality consists not of discrete objects located in space but rather of an underlying field whose interactions *produce* both objects and space" (1990:xi). The underlying common regard for the immune system in our culture allows it to become a kind of currency in which health — degrees of it — can be measured and compared among different people and populations. I will return to this point in the conclusion, but first let us look at the techniques that operate in the public domain by which we have all come to think of the body as a complex system. If the electron micrograph is one technique that scientists use to explore what makes up the body, the process to which I refer as *saturation* is one way in which the general public comes to know that the body is made up of an immune system. The term is meant to capture the sense in which awareness of and regard for the body's health as defined by the functioning of its immune system have come to be so general in the society that one cannot avoid it, wherever one turns.

In 1991, there was headline coverage of the fact that immune system dysfunctions had reached even the White House. Every member of the first family resident in the White House — Barbara Bush's Graves's disease, President Bush's Graves's disease, and their dog Millie's lupus — suffered from an autoimmune disorder (Altman 1991; "White House Water Samples" 1991). Somewhat later, major ad campaigns made direct use of the language, cells, and processes that belong to the immune system in order to promote new products. Saab, for example, promoted its chassis as "the antibody for the auto accident" (*Time*, 6 April 1992, 21).

These are just two moments in an extremely *pervasive* use of the immune system as a kind of "field" against which many phenomena have been given new interpretations and understandings. Over the course of the 1980s and 1990s, numerous long-identified conditions were redescribed as immune system dysfunctions: allergies (Davis 1989), multiple sclerosis (Thompson 1989), cancer (Squire 1987), heart disease (Braly et al. 1992), lupus (Kolata 1988), miscarriages (Brody 1992), Addison's disease, myasthenia gravis (Brownlee 1990:49), arteriosclerosis (Gates 1989), aging (Solomon et al. 1989; Foreman 1992), arthritis (Kolata 1988), and diabetes (Jewler 1989). Other, more recently identified conditions began to be understood medically as immune system dysfunctions and therefore came under wide public discussion: chronic fatigue syndrome ("You're Not Just Goldbricking" 1991), AIDS, feline immunodeficiency virus ("Three Diseases" 1992), environmental immune response (Hobbs and DeSilver 1989), idiopathic CD4+ T-lymphocytopenia (Navarro 1992), and valley fever ("Morning Edition," National Public Radio, 5 January 1993).[1]

A great many factors in a person's environment that had long been thought to influence health were explicitly reinterpreted, their effects, for good or ill, now understood to be mediated through the immune system: sunlight (Ostreicher and Klein 1987), the seasons ("Cancer and

Seasons" 1992), smoking (Diekstra 1988), silicone breast implants (Hilts 1992), electromagnetism (Brodeur 1989), radiation (Graeub 1992), chemical toxins of all kinds ("All Things Considered," National Public Radio, 15 September 1992), diet (Bialkowski 1991:16; Horwitz 1992), malnutrition ("Help May Be Too Late" 1992), exercise (deLange 1991:10), pregnancy ("Why Does the Body" 1985), fatigue (Walters 1992), consumption of cocaine ("Cocaine and Immunity" 1988), opiates (Morley et al. 1987), alcohol ("Alcohol Intake and Immunity" 1988), sleep (Moffatt 1988), academic examinations (Jemmott and Magloire 1988), and exposure to DES before birth (Brody 1993). Correlations were widely reported between the functioning of the immune system and various psychological factors: emotions (Goleman 1985), happiness (Grady 1992), depression (Brallier 1986; Roberts 1987), optimism (Goleman 1989), personality (Wood 1988), and stress (Maier and Laudenslager 1985).[2] A variety of specific social experiences were also directly related to immune function and discussed in the media. Positive effects on the immune system are claimed for confessing one's troubles (Dreher 1992), volunteering to help others (Luks 1991), caring for someone with Alzheimer's (Bower 1987), attending a support group (Goleman 1990), and becoming sexually aroused ("Sex Is the Best Cure" 1993; Kreisler 1993). Negative effects on the immune system are claimed for arguing with one's spouse (Goleman 1992), undergoing a divorce ("Divorce and Illness" 1987), and bereavement (Ornstein and Sobel 1987).

Topics in which the media had long been interested also were newly linked to immune system functioning. It was the exceptional article on cancer, organ transplants, or bone marrow transplants that did not at some point explicitly mention some aspect of the immune system. Even though it might not be mentioned in the headlines given these stories (although it often was), nevertheless the immune system frequently figured importantly in the story.[3] Descriptions of the benefits of breast milk for infants, for instance, were commonly phrased in terms of the immune system ("Keeping Breast Milk Safe" 1989).

Such reinterpretation of health in terms of immune system states was not confined to a few specialized health books and magazines. Scrutiny of the sources makes it clear that the phenomenon is widespread. In the last decade or so, articles on the immune system have appeared in such diverse publications as *Young Miss* ("Diet and Fitness" 1993), *GQ* (Heller 1988), *Vogue* (Lang 1988), *Mademoiselle* ("The Defenders" 1987), the *Christian Science Monitor* ("Defending

Children from Disease" 1979), the *Wall Street Journal* (Bishop 1988), and *Business Week* (Black 1991).

All this amounts to a change in the definition of what it means to be healthy. The immune system has moved to the very center of our culture's conception of health. How is this accomplished in these texts? Often simply by inserting the immune system into an already familiar causal series of events. For example, a broadcast of the news program "Frontline" (17 December 1992) focusing on the topic "Hunger in America" documented the extent of serious hunger statistically and elicited the audience's empathy by interviewing people struggling to feed themselves and their children. The program ended with a summary, which introduced the new causal link: these children do not die of starvation; other diseases get them first. Malnutrition weakens the immune system, and they become vulnerable to other diseases. Just as John Marcellino anticipated, attention to interior entities and processes seems to divert attention from social problems.

Coverage of the cutting edge of scientific discovery is making it increasingly clear that scientists are coming to understand the immune system as playing a central role in the body's network of causally linked systems. For example, in a finding called "extraordinary," the mechanism that links the immune system and the nervous system is revealed:

DILBERT by Scott Adams

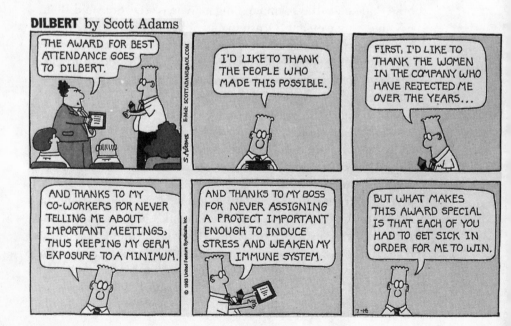

"Nerve cell endings in the skin and white blood cells of the immune system are in intimate contact, and . . . chemicals secreted by the nerves can shut down immune system cells nearby" (Kolata 1993).[4] This link explains how stress, which affects the nervous system, thus affects the immune system and can then lead directly to the onset or worsening of conditions like psoriasis and eczema. Even more recent research explains the link between sleep and the immune system: "Experiments suggest that the immune system is somehow repaired or bolstered during sleep and that it, in turn has a role in regulating sleep" (Blakeslee 1993:1). For example, the part of the mucosal immune system that lines the gut produces proteins and cytokines that can induce sleep. This explains why people feel sleepy when they are sick: the increased activity of the immune system as it fights the infection may temporarily produce more of these substances, inducing sleep while the infection lasts.

At other times, the immune system is made central to being healthy, not by making it a causal link, but simply by listing it alongside older, more familiar markers of health and well-being. A horse-racing trainer remarks of the extraordinarily successful jockey Julie Krone: "To be a great jockey, you need five traits: riding ability, physical strength, mental soundness, a great immune system, and class" (Lear 1993:38).

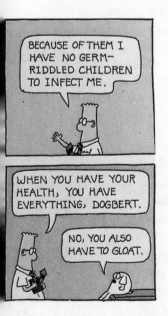

Fig. 31. *Dilbert's immune system. From C. Scott Adams,"Dilbert,"* Boston Globe, *18 July 1993. "Dilbert" reprinted by permission of UFS, Inc.*

A socially inept cartoon character, Dilbert, recites the reasons he won the award for best attendance at work: on the one hand, he has not been exposed to other people's germs because they have rejected his company, and, on the other, his immune system has not been stressed because his boss never gives him an important job (see fig. 31).

Other reports use more elaborate techniques. In *The Healing Power of Doing Good*, Allan Luks supports his claim that volunteering to help others boosts the immune system by surveying 3,300 volunteers, of whom 3,296 responded (Luks 1991:7–8). The survey results showed that, "of the 95 percent of respondents who reported the sensations of helper's high, nine out of ten rated their health as better than others their age" (p. 81). Luks's own research, with its large numbers and statistical correlations, is then buttressed by reference to authorities who did related studies in psychoneuroimmunology: for example, Robert Ader, who showed that rats could be conditioned to suppress their immune systems; and David McClelland, who demonstrated increases in immune system function after subjects had watched a film about Mother Teresa aiding the sick and dying. Finally, visual evidence is presented: David and Susan Feltens "actually photographed the connections between nerve endings and white blood cells that fight off infection. This was another landmark in the effort to prove that the mind and the immune system are able to talk to each other." All this evidence, including his own, is marshaled by Luks to demonstrate that "our immune system 'knows' how we think and feel and is affected by our general mental state — and, in circular fashion, can affect it as well" (pp. 86, 83).

Other studies produce immediate physical evidence using tests that reveal the contents of body substances (blood samples) immediately following instances of the two events that the authors claim are causally linked. In one case, the physical evidence proves a link between confession and a stronger immune system:

> The research team [headed by James Pennebaker] drew blood from the study participants before and after the writing exercise [in which subjects wrote about "the most upsetting or traumatic experience" of their entire lives] and again six weeks later. They focused on one important measure: the activity of the subjects' T cells when exposed to foreign agents. . . . Compared to students in the control group, those who wrote about traumas showed a marked increase in the liveliness of their T cells after the exercise.

Moreover, students who confided traumas that they had previously held back from telling others (called "high disclosers") had the most conspicuous upsurge in T cell activity. (Dreher 1992:78)

In another case, the physical evidence produced by blood tests proves a link between marital fights and weakened immune systems. In this study, ninety couples were brought into a laboratory and asked to resolve an issue on which they disagreed. Continuous blood monitoring for twenty-four hours allowed their immune responses to be measured during and after the discussion. "We found a far stronger effect on the couples' immune system than we ever expected," said Dr. Kiecolt-Glaser. "Those couples who had most hostility and negativity during the discussions showed a drop on eight immune measures for the next 24 hours. The more hostile you are during a marital argument, the harder it is on your immune system" (Goleman 1992:1). Plainer evidence of the pressure for *harmony* arising out of concern for the health of the immune system could not be found.

These studies are making visible — either literally, through photographs of the microscopic process, or putatively, through the results of blood tests — a new causal linkage that makes the immune system central to our definition of health and how it might be achieved or maintained. Describing the impact of Pasteur's making the microbe visible in his laboratory, Bruno Latour writes:

Pasteur adds to all the forces that composed French society at the time a new force for which he is the only credible spokesman — the microbe. You cannot build economic relations without this "tertium quid" since the microbe, if unknown, can bitter your beer, spoil your wine, make the mother of your vinegar sterile, bring back cholera with your goods, or kill your factotum sent to India. You cannot build a hygienist social movement without it, since no matter what you do for the poor masses crowded in shanty towns, they will still die if you do not control this invisible agent. . . . A group of people, equipped with a laboratory — the only place where the invisible agent is made visible — will easily be situated everywhere in all these relations, wherever the microbe can be seen to intervene. (Latour 1983:157)

Speaking from the vantage point of the 1990s, we could say that the immune system can translate sunlight into sickness, optimism into health. It can make those who volunteer healthy and those who do not confess sick. It can kill malnourished children before starvation does. It can attack our very bones, nerves, and organs. If we do not understand it, we may be unable to transplant organs and bone marrow, graft tissue, or infuse blood. If we do not understand it, we will not be able to develop vaccines to protect our population against the new highly mutable viruses like HIV and Ebola emerging from disrupted ecosystems.

Latour's study of Pasteur traces how Pasteur extended the conditions of the laboratory into the society beyond it. The psychoneuroimmunologic studies mentioned above seem to do this also: submit the everyday events of fights between spouses or writing down experiences to laboratory conditions so that they can be controlled, measured, graphed, and correlated with immune functions. In addition, studies by Luks and others contain within them recipes for taking individual action, to put these newly emerging truths about the immune system to work in daily life. One encourages us to use its "guidelines for a written confession" in order to carry out "psychic preventive maintenance" (Dreher 1992:80). Luks includes a chapter on "getting started" followed by an appendix with hundreds of addresses and phone numbers of local and national volunteer organizations (Luks 1991). Moreover, many media articles and books contain a plethora of recipes for specific tonics, remedies, and self-improvement programs: eat garlic (Murray 1990:12), Chinese astragulus (McCaleb 1990:22), a combination of many herbs and mushrooms (Hobbs and DeSilver 1989:72); don't eat too much fat (Heller 1988); exercise in careful moderation (Laliberte 1992:56; LaForge 1989); tailor your diet (Brody 1989); practice relaxation and biofeedback (Larsen 1985); use light therapy (Gilbert 1992).

Inevitably, given the omnipresent commodification of health in U.S. culture, stores now provide plenty of health-enhancing products intended specifically to help people protect their immune systems. The Baltimore area stocks a sample: "immune fitness tea," recipes for "immune soup," "Immunergy, Fuel for Life in the Fast Lane," "Advanced Defense System Plus." More expensive items (from the 1992 Selfcare catalog) include "Home Bright Light III" ($499) to combat seasonal depression or a "Dust Mite-Hunter Vacuum" ($369). This vacuum uses three filters to trap dust mites and then destroys them in the heat from the exhaust: the mite, identified as "Microscopic Dermatophagoides Pteranysimus . . . far too ugly to show," can trigger many allergic reactions and asthma. Recalling the discussion of electron micrographs in Chapter 8, an ad for an inexpensive version of the vacuum in *American Health* (November 1992, 20) does not hesitate to show its readers a micrograph of the dust mite, ugly as some may find it. Note that, despite its association with dust, the dust mite is not something, like the germs of the 1940s and 1950s, that can be simply cleaned away. Nor does it operate like a germ. It is an allergen, and only those with overly sensitive immune systems need bother about it.

In the late twentieth century, then, most of us are commonly, and constantly, taking account of the effects of everyday activities on our immune systems (with or without the help of special products).

Not only is awareness of the immune system *pervasive*, however; it is also *extended* from the primarily visual media discussed so far into other realms of sensory experience. There are many routes through which knowledge about the immune system is being transmitted viscerally. Perhaps most astounding of all is the amusement park ride "Body Wars," which attendants told us is by far the most popular exhibit at Epcot Center near Disney World in Florida.[5] In a coming to life of the movie *The Fantastic Voyage*, the ride is a multisensory experience that creates the illusion of being miniaturized in order to travel through the body of a volunteer, a twelve-year-old boy, to "actually see the immune system in action," contending with a splinter and a bruise.

Possibly more significant than "Body Wars," in terms of its impact on great numbers of people in a variety of nations, is the educational material developed by the Jerusalem AIDS Project in Israel. This material, published in Hebrew, English, German, and Spanish, contains curriculum outlines, color slides, and specific suggestions for games to teach children through play how their immune systems work: groups of children can pretend to be the various cells of the immune system and then dramatically act out the ways in which they interact (Schenker 1988, 1992). An electronic version of a similar idea is contained in a software program called "The Immune System" (marketed by Marshware in 1990). The program provides a game of checkers between germs and phagocytes in which the child must answer questions about the immune system correctly in order to move pieces about the board (Phenix 1992).[6] Inevitably, experiential workshops are also beginning to appear, which will allow people to explore and enhance the relations between their emotional states, sensuality, and sexuality and their immune systems.[7]

To express the effect of money on societies in which it circulated, Marx makes the point that the labor produced by a farmer, miner, or weaver is each different in kind until money enters as a medium in which worth can be measured in the same coin.[8] Is the immune system functioning with respect to the body in the same sort of way?[9] Are we seeing the development of a "health currency" in terms of which exceedingly diverse and widely ranging forces and causes affecting health can be measured in the same coin?

As I was at the point of asking myself this question, I realized that the "saturation" of our ideas about health had to be incomplete because one major set of health problems does not seem to be pervaded by immune system thinking: heart diseases.[10] The popular press has not yet put heart disease in an immune system framework — the heart is still a mechanical pump with wires and pipes that can burn out or become clogged. But there are signs of an imminent change. Hypertension, often implicated in heart disease, is frequently linked to stress in media accounts, and, as we have seen, stress is solidly linked to the immune system. I consulted with medical researchers knowledgeable about both immunology and cardiology, who told me that the connections between heart disease and the immune system are only now beginning to be seen.[11] Reading the sources that they mentioned, I found that emerging research is suggesting that the lesions of atherosclerosis (hardening of the arteries) may represent immune or autoimmune responses (Ross 1990; Libby et al. 1989; Libby and Hansson 1991; Clerc 1991). A short time later, I found that the major science journal *Nature* had just published a lengthy review article in which the complex connections between the activities of the immune system and atherosclerosis is explored at length (Ross 1993). The field of health is not yet completely saturated with immune system thinking, but it seems likely that even the quintessential mechanical body part, the heart, will soon succumb as well.

Estimates are only now beginning to appear in literature relatively accessible to the general public that describe numerically how extensive immune dysfunction would be if heart disease were implicated: "Five percent of adults in Europe and North America — two thirds of them women — suffer from an autoimmune disease, many from more than one at a time. The affected population may turn out to be far larger if, as some workers suspect, autoimmunity plays an important secondary role in atherosclerosis, the cause of half the deaths in the Western world" (Steinman 1993:107).

CHAPTER 10

Educating and Training the Body: Vaccines and Tests

I want to say: an education quite different from ours might also be the foundation for quite different concepts.
LUDWIG WITTGENSTEIN, *Zettel*

According to the *Oxford English Dictionary*, *immune* originally meant to be exempt from the requirement of service to the state. It was not until the late nineteenth century that the entity that the "immune" individual could ward off became not the state but disease. The two meanings of the word came together when immunization was developed and made available to the public, often without choice, through resources and personnel mobilized by the state and the medical profession. Although people often assume that vaccination is beneficial — indeed, the Clinton administration seeks to make vaccination a universal right — we will find that not everyone thinks that vaccination is a good thing. Accepting vaccination means accepting the state's power to impose a particular view about the body and its immune system — the view developed by medical science. To understand how the practice of vaccination becomes established in society (or fails to), we need to examine more closely a key feature of the way in which the immune system is understood scientifically.

In immunology, as it is understood in research contexts, and as it is presented in the popular media, the links among the parts of the immune system are often described as lines of communication. In our interviews, people (scientists as well as nonscientists; see fig. 32) generally see the immune system as being held together by the messages that are communicated among its parts. What determines whether this communication is effective are such matters as "recognition"/"misrecognition," "memory"/"forgetting," and "knowledge"/"ignorance." Most of the time, the immune system "recognizes" or "identifies" things that are a threat to the body's health and "knows" what to do in response. Sometimes this is because it "remembers" the threat from "seeing" it previously (Brackette Thompson) and having "learned" about it then.

Since the immune system is thought of as a community of sentient "beings" who remember and forget, it makes sense, especially in the American context, that people readily think of this community in terms of the model of a liberal democracy, in which education plays an important role in allowing its members to achieve their potential. The thymus is often described as the school or college of the immune system, where T cells are educated. Here is how one of my immunology professors described the thymus in a graduate class:

> The thymus doesn't filter anything. It's got a very different function. It's a nursery. It's a T cell nursery. T cells, cells coming from the bone marrow, come into the thymus, settle there, mature, get their antigen receptors, learn who they are, whatever that means. They learn whether they are cytoxin T cells or helper T cells, and then another amazing thing happens to the thymus. And these cells that capture antigen receptors that somehow are programmed to react against self protein get eliminated in the thymus — before they leave the thymus they get killed. How that happens we don't know. But about 95 percent of the cells that enter the thymus never leave. They mature there, but they are recognized as a danger to the body, and they get killed, right

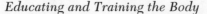

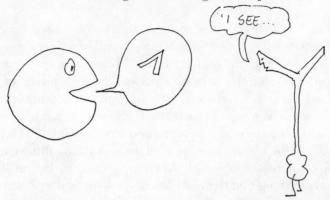

Fig. 32. *Umberto Eco's "doodle" of an antibody talking to a cell at the conference on the semiotics of the immune system. From E. E. Sercarz et al., eds.,* The Semiotics of Cellular Communication in the Immune System *(1988:207).*

> there in the thymus. Only a small percentage of mature cells leave. Another amazing thing about the thymus is that it is very large in the newborn and it starts getting smaller at about the teenage years and then in the adult it is quite small. So the thymus that's sitting above the heart between the lungs is quite large. In contrast, the adult thymus just looks like a twisted rod, and it has almost lost its function. All the T cells that have been educated . . . while you were a newborn or while you were young are now fed out to lymph nodes and spleen and have already learned who they are and who they are going to react to. So that in the adult thymus there isn't much T cell education going on anymore. T cells can survive outside of the bone marrow. They survive in the lymph node. (Richard Walton)

A harsh school indeed, in which only 5 percent graduate and the rest are killed![1]

A medical scientist explains the time that T cells spend in the thymus as their apprenticeship:

> Well, the immune system is sort of a blind system of recognition that you need to teach. So it's able to recognize anything, including things that don't even exist now. And the basis of self versus nonself discrimination is that the universe has billions of billions of billions of shapes and all sorts of molecules that could potentially be harmful to your body, and your body contains 1 billion

shapes, who knows. And you have to classify. . . . You have to be able to tell the system what is the self and what is the rest of the universe. And, as the system starts going, you go through an apprenticeship that is in the fetus and the early phases of childhood, and . . . maybe even through your entire life you keep learning about self versus nonself. Essentially, you tell a system that's able to recognize anything and attack anything, This is your body—don't touch it. And, if there is anything different from that, you react against [it]. When the system works fine, if some foreign thing that the body has never seen during this apprenticeship time, if one of these antigens occurs, whether it's a bacteria or virus or even a totally new chemical molecule that a chemist just synthesized [that] is being injected into your body, the system will react against it and try to reject it. And when the system breaks down, either it does not recognize the nonself, which means that you cannot build any immune response against an attack from outside, or it stops recognizing things that actually are self and attacks that. So that's an autoimmune disease. So how does it work? Actually, I don't know, and I don't think anybody really knows. [Laughs.] (Ken Holden)

In his article on the immune system for Encyclopedia Britannica's *Great Ideas Today, 1991*, Michael Edidin elaborates the educational functions of the thymus. Occasionally, he tells us, some growing cells, "the clever but thuggish teenagers of the population, manage to smuggle anti-'self' receptors out of their school and into circulation. Like some teenagers, they have not thought about the future and do not quite know what faces them." If these cells respond wrongly to "self," they will be paralyzed for life and never be able to respond to anything again. Having eluded the first test of their schooling, these cells are condemned "to life in solitude when [they] fail [their] second test against 'self'" (Edidin 1991:44).[2]

Even immune system cells that do not emerge from the thymus are "educated." B cells are "educated" in the bone marrow, where they learn incredible specificity (Dwyer 1988:47). One children's book about the immune system organizes its story line around the immature cells in the bone marrow going to school ("RubroSchool" for the red cells and "LeukoSchool" for the white cells) until they have learned enough to carry out their functions in the body (Benziger 1989). Vaccinations play their role in this world as special courses, a designer education for the (usually) young immune system. The vaccine gives the immune system a kind of postthymus and postmarrow course in recognizing a disease organism (small pox, diphtheria, polio, or whatever).

In our interviews, some people explain how they understand vaccines as training or educating the immune system:

> *What's your conception of how a vaccine works?*
> It's a form of the disease itself, it's a very weak form, so that the antibodies in your system can I guess be introduced to it, interact with it, and conquer it as it were, so that your system can now go, Oh, OK, I know what this is. I know it doesn't belong here. And the antibodies kind of go, This doesn't belong here, whop! Let's, you know, get rid of it. We recognize this as something that is foreign to the body, that doesn't belong here. (Paul Silverstein)

> *OK, go ahead. What's your idea of how a vaccine works?*
> I think my most basic idea of how a vaccine works is that you put some dead or severely disabled germs, bad things, bacteria or viruses, into your body that in and of themselves do not pose a threat to disable you. And that your body sends again these little white blood cells to come and check 'em out, and they have some kind of a struggle with them, but they learn, through their struggle, what these bad things are about, so that . . . the next time they chance upon something like this, they're going to have no problem coping with it. (Eliot Green)

> *Let's say you've just gotten a measles vaccination. Sort of sketch out the little play. What's going on in your body? Imagine what building up resistance looks like. How is your body doing it?*
> OK. Back to our little soldiers, the soldiers march around the body trying to keep things cool, you know, and then they like encounter this new species, and it's like, Oh shit! We don't know anything about this guy. What are we going to do? Wait, wait, wait, wait, we've got a little bit of an advantage here, you know. *This* is just a small amount of *that*, you know. [There's] a lot of us, and we don't know about them, but, you know, maybe we can take them, you know, and let's like send our little spies or whatever and try to figure out what it's all about, what we

can do to fight it, and that type of thing. You know, I think that's
kind of the way it works. (Charles Kingsley)

Vaccines "introduce" new information in a simple (weak) form that
allows the immune system to "learn," "figure out what it's all about" in
a training exercise. Many people had heard about the recommendation to be revaccinated for measles and explained the need by saying
that the immune system might have forgotten what it once knew and
need to be reintroduced to something that it could no longer recognize (Michael Spicer, Mary Loran).

    If vaccines are seen as a form of "education" for the immune sys-
tem, it does not follow that everyone will desire this "education."
Sometimes people feel reluctant to accept vaccination, even in the face
of government regulations that make it compulsory for school attendance. Sometimes people refuse vaccinations for themselves or their
children and suffer the consequences.[3] It is as if people are saying to
the state as purveyor of health education, and of education for the
immune system (in the form of a vaccination), Thanks anyway, but my
immune system and I will learn to adjust to our environment ourselves.
As Katherine Johnson put it, "I have real mixed feelings about things
like immunizations and flu shots and stuff like that." She refused to
give her son vaccinations in infancy but finally did, "mostly because I
didn't want to have to deal with fighting schools forever, and I couldn't
prove like religious or medical reasons not to. But I really think that,
again in medicine, we use overkill and that sometimes we use overkill
even when the consequences of that maybe outweigh the benefits. . . .
I just don't trust medicine." As for herself, "I will probably never take
a flu shot as long as I live. Like what is the point? That's my point. What
is the point? Give me the flu to keep me from getting the flu? OK, fine.
You know what I mean? So [heavy with sarcasm] — whatever you say."

    The deeper reason for her reluctance goes "back to the immune sys-
tem." Only when "there's a breakdown in your immune system" do you
"get sick." Even in the face of "bugs" from our global travel or pollution, "there's a whole lot of things that we just walk around with and
manage until we break down, and so I'm not so sure that we need to
run around and get immunized against them all." Zoh Hieronimus, the
founder of Ruscombe Mansion, a Baltimore community health center
for alternative healing, takes time on her local radio talk show to make
her feelings clear about the Clinton plan to increase funding for vacci-

nation of the country's children: "'At two months old, let's shoot our babies full of poison,' she modestly proposes, oozing sarcasm and sublimated fury" (Shapiro 1993:1).

To begin to get a deeper understanding of this kind of reluctance, consider the way in which an M.D. who practices nutritional medicine explains it. What he makes clear is the fear that vaccines will harm the immune system, leading to various kinds of immune-compromised states:

> There's two major factors that have occurred in modern society — severe pollution and vaccinating human beings, routine vaccination of humans — both of which can have severe effects on the immune system. And I don't know which is which, but, you know, there are cases of chronic fatigue syndrome occurring immediately after rubella vaccine, for example. You know, we're pumpin' this polio vaccine and DPT and whatever else we're givin' kids.
> *So you don't think that vaccines are very healthy for individuals?*
> I don't know. . . . Now, all these new opportunistic infections that are occurring. We've got this controversial syndrome called "the yeast connection," or Candida-related complex. It was only described fourteen years ago. And I get, you know, dozens and dozens of people coming in all the time with that. There's the Epstein-Barr virus, or chronic fatigue syndrome, which is new. No more than ten or twelve years old. You've got AIDS, which is ten or twelve years old. You've got herpes simplex, which has become a bigger epidemic than it ever was. So there's something that's happened to us. And the two things that I can think of, the pollution and the vaccines. I can't think anything else. Maybe somebody else can.
> *Yeah.*
> I mean, if you inject a foreign antigen into somebody to raise the antibody levels, we have no idea what the long-term consequences of that are.
> *Yeah. So it's a little bit naive to think that it has no side effect?*
> Right. Well, we know that pertussis, in some cases, causes neurotoxicity. But in terms of the long term, I mean, we've got

more lupus, we've got multiple sclerosis, we've got more cancer, we've got all these diseases that I mentioned. Asthma has doubled in frequency in the past ten years.
But of course you can argue that we have better tools for diagnosing those diseases.
It's not hard to diagnose multiple sclerosis. It's pretty obvious. And cancer is becoming more severe and common.
But you think that it's the environment, the lifestyle, and therefore nutrition, too, then.
Sure, absolutely. (Martin Rabinow)

A nurse elaborates a similar theme:

> I'm not so sure that disease is a bad thing. I'm not so sure that the vaccine is not a bad thing either because there isn't really that much that's known about the immune system, from what I've read, and so. . . . There's a theory that says that there are only a limited, I don't know that much about immunology, but there are only, say, a limited amount of antibodies that can respond to a given disease, so if you use up all those antibodies from vaccines, then whenever they're really needed, they're taken up with something else, in other words, they become specific for one disease only. Which makes sense. . . .
> *So what do you think about the teenagers having a measles vaccination?*
> I'm against vaccines altogether, and since they've started this MMR vaccine, there are a lot of teenagers that are coming down with measles and mumps, after being vaccinated, and they get a lot sicker than they would have if they had those diseases when they were children. . . . I've just come to question everything, and vaccines in particular, and I feel like medicine in this country has become almost like a religion, that's sanctioned by the government. Vaccines are not a voluntary thing. They're something that are required by law to have your children immunized. And I just feel like that's taking away from, that there should be freedom of choice. (Laura Peterson)

A popular book about the hazards of immunization puts concern about vaccines and the immune system together with measures that anyone can take to stay healthy without vaccines:

Our immune system has a built-in intelligence, always correcting, altering course based on individual needs and conditions. It would be wise to start trusting the immune system, rather than assuming it is inferior until artificially "immunized." . . . Taking full responsibility for the condition of the individual human body opens the door to better health. Through this awareness and acceptance, one can see that illness is simply a matter of how susceptible the body is made. One can make choices in his life that either prepares him for disease or builds for health. (Cournoyer 1991:11, 104)

The idea that one can train one's own immune system in various ways is expressed commonly in our interviews and is hardly confined to health purists. A college student we interviewed said that, during their twenty years together, she and her immune system have gotten used to each other: "It's gotten used to my way of living. My lack of sleep, and my bad eating habits, it's sort of grown to accept it because I'm not sick the entire school year, but I hardly sleep the entire school year, and I don't eat right. If I were to get a new immune system, then I would be sick the entire school year until I had it trained that this is me and this is how I function, so help me out a little bit" (Elizabeth Able).

In American society, education and training are almost always part of processes of social differentiation (who goes to what schools, for how long, with what result).[4] It was no surprise, then, to find that education and training in the body also produced social differentiation. The basic message (which I came across in many contexts) is that immune systems are not created equal. In Edidin's encyclopedia article: "Vaccination always carries a slight risk, because there are always unknown factors in the process. Though the vaccine is thoroughly tested and as pure as possible, the people who are to be vaccinated are an uncontrolled lot varying in their genetic makeup, their health, and the quality of their immune systems. This means that every so often vaccination brings on an unpleasant reaction" (Edidin 1991:49). An interview with an acupuncturist opposed to any vaccines gives the opposite point of view about the value of vaccines but the same point of view about variation in the quality of people's immune systems: "I tend to believe that, you know, measles, this, that, and the other — all these different vaccines, if people don't have a good lifestyle or a living standard, they're very helpful, but aside from that, for most of the middle-class and upper-class people, [they are] total nonsense, and they're just asking for much more trouble, you know. They leave the body filled with inactive pathogens to clog it up that are eventually going to change somehow the chemistry" (Barry Folsom). His point is that the "well-brought-up" immune system already knows most of what it needs to know and that, even though it is being continually exposed to new pathogens, it is overkill to keep bombarding it with unneeded information.

Despite variation in the population, from people with superior immune systems, superbly trained and continuously reeducated to respond flexibly to any new circumstance in the environment, to people with slow, rigid, inflexible immune systems, there is one contemporary threat that, once ensconced, defeats almost everyone's immune system: HIV. One problem that HIV poses to the immune system of those who are infected is the same problem that it poses to those who would develop a vaccine: the virus changes its form so rapidly (hypermutating) that it escapes both the efforts of the immune system to catch it and the effects of any vaccine. The combatants are, on the one side, a virus that is "smarter than we are" because it mutates with remarkable speed (Creedon 1992) and, on the other side, only hope: for a vaccine that can "teach the immune system how to stop HIV" (Cohen 1992:152).[5] Since "history has shown that it is extremely difficult to develop protective vaccines against organisms that can mutate quickly and present constantly changing antigens to the immune system," our only hope for the present is to rely on public education (Anderson and May 1993). Thus, ironically, the present inability of a vaccine to "educate" the immune system about HIV forces us to rely on education of a different kind.

People who decide that they want to avoid the system of "state education" for their immune systems (vaccines) and develop their own "private schooling" instead are not so much "resisting" vaccination as they are developing a positive view of what their health is. This view shares with immunology the basic notion of the body as a training ground for the immune system, but it denies the benefits of crash courses. Such people may have been engaging in a lifetime of preparation, training and nurturing their immune systems through diet, exercise, avoiding stress, and other healthy practices. They may quite reasonably believe that they and their immune systems are already able to change and adapt flexibly, rapidly responding as needed to a continuously changing environment. In such a view, a vaccine, bludgeoning the delicate adjustment of the finely tuned immune system with antigens at a time when there is no actual threat, could easily be seen as something undermining health.[6]

It is important to note the juxtaposition between the agile person with his or her constantly adapting immune system, on the one hand, and the rigid, unthinking, unchanging state on the other. As we saw in Chapter 7, old-style bureaucratic governments are the paradigm of ossified, rule-bound, inflexible, cumbersome, sluggish organizations (Osborne and Gaebler 1992:12). A vaccine policy administered in the style of such a government could be expected to share these characteristics: it would not be able to discriminate among individuals according to their particular health needs; it would not be able to respond very much to the particular circumstances of any single child. Karen Plummer, who now has serious second thoughts about state requirements for vaccination before a child can enter school, came to these doubts because her third child has leukemia. She told me that she thought that his early childhood vaccinations might have impaired his immune system and helped cause his cancer: "Given how sensitive he had been since birth, I knew I should never have let him be vaccinated. He was too pure."

In our research we found reluctance to vaccinate across age, gender, ethnic, and class lines. When one looks at the pattern of who in the population actually gets vaccinated from the perspective of a public health expert, however, it would be clear that many more middle-class than poor, inner-city parents obtain early vaccinations for their children (DeParle 1993). There are doubtless many reasons for this, including differences in income, availability of health insurance, level of education, availability of transportation, motivation, and so on. Despite such overall patterns, however, some people at every income and education level do question the value of vaccination as a public good.

IN ADDITION to vaccination, there are other procedures related to the immune system — including tests or measures of immune function — that people can do themselves, or have a doctor do, regularly, to monitor the state of their immune functions. This kind of monitoring goes on very frequently in relation to the functioning of the heart: consider how many people know their blood pressure or serum cholesterol levels. With respect to the immune system, these personal monitoring practices are only beginning. In my research, I found every variety of reaction to testing for HIV. There was my own fear of being tested, on the one hand, and there was the widespread resistance to compulsory HIV testing in the AIDS activist community, resistance based on privacy and civil rights issues. But there was also nearly uniform agreement among the injectable drug users we interviewed that compulsory testing would be a good thing. Since they already find themselves tested often — in their frequent encounters with the prison system — compulsory testing of the general population would make them feel as if they were treated more equally.[7]

People who know that they are HIV+ and symptomatic with AIDS become rapidly drawn into regular testing of their immune functions and can often talk exceedingly knowledgeably, especially about their T cell level. My first buddy, Mark Scott, was very aware of measures of his immune function. Everything depended, in his eyes, on having a high enough T cell count to justify a bone marrow transplant from his identical twin. But even Mark could find medical reliance on testing oppressive, bringing him as it did into close proximity with some of the disturbing heterosexual body models of biomedicine.

This became clear when Mark was presented at "grand rounds," the elaborate, formal presentations of cases held in a large hospital lecture hall. Although Mark was extremely ill, recovering from a serious toxoplasmosis infection, he was elated at the prospect of being presented at grand rounds. He told me the week before that he was the one and only patient his doctor, Dr. Walker, wanted to present. He said that he was going to try to get across the need for a patient to be responsible for his own illness, no matter how sick. He wanted to convey the importance of not taking a doctor's word for it and of learning as much as possible by asking questions. He was planning to start off with a funny but risqué joke, "so that they could see I have a sense of humor." When he told me this, he was in the hospital, unable to walk or even to sit up. Three days later — by dint of incredible determination — he was shaved, with a fresh haircut, dressed in a dark double-breasted suit, leaning on the arm of Dr. Walker walking across the stage at grand rounds.

Far from beginning with a joke, Mark had to respond to a series of detailed questions put to him by Dr. Walker, in which the various stages of his disease were constructed entirely in terms of the progressive elimination of T 4 cells:

Mr. Scott has an identical twin, and he underwent a series of leukocyte infusions from the identical twin, followed by bone marrow transplantation. Before the bone marrow transplantation, do you know what the status of your immune system was?

[Mark Scott replies,] Yes I do.

What was it?

My T 4 count was 60.

60. OK. The normal value at that laboratory was 600, 800? So you had less than 10 percent of the normal number of helper T cells. Had you had that test done before?

[Mr. Scott looks puzzled.]

The T cell count, before you went to NIH.

In 1984 it was normal.

So over a period of three or four years, the helper T cells, the primary target of HIV, had fallen from near normal, a near normal range, down to a very low range of a T 4 count of 60. What happened with bone marrow transplantation?

I believe to this day that I got a boost. I was very strong for a while after the bone marrow. I went back to college and studied word processing and was making a 4 point while working a full-time job. Only in the last six months was I ill.

And in terms of the laboratory evaluations that they did . . . clearly functionally you did extremely well. You were working full time, functioning entirely normally. The laboratory tests that they did to monitor you, what did that show?

[Mr. Scott shakes his head uncomprehendingly.]

The T cells, did they change?

My T cells went up after the bone marrow to about 180 and stayed there for about three months before coming back down to 60.

So there was a transient *increase in your helper T cells, but functionally you felt fine.*

Mark's condition is relentlessly defined by his T 4 cell count, despite his "functioning" well in school, work, etc. In this process, given the significance of T 4 cells as virile, heterosexual heroes in the armamentarium of the body, Mark is defined as impotent and feeble. The force of this drama could not have struck deeper when, later, many doctors came down onto the stage to congratulate Mark and his doctor: they said that Mark's presence had "given AIDS a human face." As far as Mark's experience went, grand rounds had given his AIDS a face he could no longer recognize. Mark and other HIV+ people I knew were caught in a double bind by their reliance on tests of their immune function. Mark wanted to know the results of his tests but did not want to be defined by those tests.

The general population of the United States is only beginning to demand the extension of tests of immune function. Knowledge about how to get the information that such tests can provide still has a kind of underground existence. *Prevention Magazine's 30 Day Plan to Super Immunity* reveals the crucial information: the next time you have a routine blood test, look at the lab slip. Multiply the number marked "percent of lymphocytes" by the number marked "white count." This will give you the number of lymphocytes per millimeter of blood. Then you can record the level and watch for any change over time (Michaud and Feinstein 1989:369). Should such knowledge become extended widely and people come to know their lymphocyte count as readily as they know their blood pressure, we will have entered a new phase in the interactions between popular concepts of the immune system and scientific techniques to monitor it.

CHAPTER 11

Educating and Training at Work[1]

Learning is dramatic and it's quick.... When you get people off the ground, they're scared. It's an unnatural place for humans to be. We're not squirrels."

KIMBERLY LEEMAN

Analysts and writers of widely different political persuasions currently agree that the global economic condition has recently changed dramatically. In Part II, we saw how political economists characterize these changes, and the broad outlines of their characterizations match those of other observers across the political spectrum. In the words of Rosabeth Moss Kantor, a professor at the Harvard Business School and a consultant to many Fortune 500 companies, the dominance of the "large twentieth-century corporation based on mass-production, mechanical technologies favoring routinized jobs, and American economic hegemony" is giving way "as other nations come to the fore, as the global marketplace and international competition expand, as technology becomes more complex and more rapidly changing, as women and minorities seek access to the better jobs, and as growth slows (or reverses) in traditional industries" (1989:306).

In order to survive in this changed environment, a wide variety of human resource managers, consultants, and authors are advocating that American corporations must become like biological systems that successfully survive in nature. Following "nature's templates," the corporation must become a "learning organization," that is, an organization that is "continually expanding its capacity to create its future" (Senge 1990:14). In a book called *Grow or Die* that executives in a major multinational corporation told me had crucially formed their recent thinking, we hear: "The first postulate of transformation states that *human behavior has naturally evolved from biological behavior*, and that the behavior of all living things is *growth-directed* activity. The mandate of nature, as we observe it on every hand, is the same — 'grow or die'" (Ainsworth-Land 1986:12). As cells, organisms, and organizations evolve, they must pass through levels of growth, from accretive growth (self-expansion), to replicative growth (self-duplication), to mutual growth (sexual fusion and recombination). The injunction to *grow* means to grow in complexity and interdependence, not simply in size:

> As a society, we now balance ourselves between eight thousand years of competitive, second-phase growing and the emergent cooperative, third-phase growth characteristic of our own development. . . . We struggle with "wholing" as we try to become whole persons with a whole-world consciousness. This "wholistic" consciousness will force us to recognize and integrate those parts of ourselves — male/female identities, left/right brains, divergent/convergent thinking — that we have long neglected while striving for a strong sense of "self." Societally we feel the pressures of integrating long-ignored portions of our population — women, minorities, handicapped. As part of an emergent world community, we experience the impact of the reality that we are all in this together. (Ainsworth-Land 1986:xi–xii)

Each person will have to become transformed as a part of the growth process, as fundamentally as when a caterpillar becomes a butterfly:

Change in our times is a given. The responsibility for continued
and creative leadership is a must. We must shift the executive
mind-set from "How do we survive?" to "How can we thrive?"
given the challenge of keeping the organization alive, healthy and
innovative over time. "What the caterpillar calls the end of the
world, the master calls the butterfly" (Richard Bach, *Illusions*).
(Rockford Co. materials)

This growth entails a reconceptualization of boundaries: "We tend
to blame outside circumstances for our problems. 'Someone else' —
the competitors, the press, the changing mood of the marketplace, the
government — did it to us. Systems thinking shows us that there is no
outside; that you and the cause of your problems are part of a single
system" (Senge 1990:67). Concretely, this means that corporations are
admonished to make links across all kinds of divisions, both within the
corporation and among different companies: "Lean, agile . . . companies can stretch in three ways. They can *pool* resources with others, *ally*
to exploit an opportunity, or *link* systems in a partnership. In short they
can become better 'PALs' with other organizations — from venture
collaborators to suppliers, service contractors, and even unions"
(Kantor 1989:118). Tom Peters cites an example that illustrates why
these linkages are increasingly necessary: "A piece of ice hockey equipment, designed in Scandinavia, engineered in the U.S. to meet the
requirements of the large U.S. and Canadian market, manufactured in
Korea and distributed through a multinational market network with
initial distribution from Japan. *The question is: Where is, what is the
organization?*" (Miles quoted in Peters 1992:149). The answer is, Not
where or what we have been accustomed to. The preeminent model
of industrial organization of the decades before 1970, which has been
called "Fordist," has undergone *radical* revision. Gone is the linear
work sequence of the moving assembly line, its machinery dedicated
to mass production and mass marketing. Instead, the organization is a
fleeting, fluid network of alliances, a highly decoupled and dynamic
form with great organizational flexibility.

Two human resource managers discussed the differences involved
in being part of a company that has made such linkages:

CARY NELSON: From a new person's perspective, having been in
personnel for five or six years, this is really more challenging

because you are forced to broaden your scope. To think and act group as opposed to think and act for strictly individuals. *Individually?*

LAURA GERSHON: And so I mean it's a real challenge. This is not the way I've done it before, but it's that little excitement inside 'cause your own boundaries get broken.

CN: Laura taught me through a model of concentric circles where you go from the individual to the other individual to another, then to the group, then to the organization, then to the community out in the whole. That's the working model that she likes to use, and I can see how it functions. It also is in keeping with an ancient Buddhist prayer that a peaceful person makes a peaceful family, a peaceful family makes a peaceful community, a peaceful community makes a peaceful city, a peaceful city makes a peaceful state, a peaceful state makes a peaceful country, a peaceful country makes a peaceful nation, a peaceful nation makes a peaceful world.

But simply making new linkages is not enough. To compete successfully in the "corporate olympics" (Kantor 1989:18), corporate bodies must become agile (p. 28), leaner (p. 294), in shape (p. 67), flexible enough to change (p. 89). Like the human body, American *corporate* bodies that are healthy are "focused, fast, friendly and flexible" (p. 361). Successful corporations will "combine the power of a giant with the agility of a dancer" (p. 33). To survive, corporations will have to be "fluid, ever shifting in size, shape, and arrangement" (Peters 1992:147).

These prescriptions are being made by a wide variety of management specialists who have embraced a way of thinking about reorganizing the work process that we have already met briefly — total quality management, or TQM for short.[2] Although the central concepts of TQM have been present in the business literature for more than a decade, President Clinton has now given this school of thought a national forum, surrounding himself with people like Robert Reich and Donna Shalala who have been advocating principles associated with TQM for some time.[3]

TQM advocates are far from a unified group; within their ranks are proponents of many different approaches to the reorganization of the workforce.[4] When I first came upon TQM from within my sheltered position as a college professor, I naively assumed that it was an arcane school of thought with a limited impact. I have since learned otherwise.

TQM is embraced widely as the most effective way forward out of the economic troubles that the United States is experiencing (no fewer than three issues of *Business Week* had special sections on or were devoted *entirely* to TQM in 1991–92 [see Port 1992]).[5] It is actively developed by a number of large professional associations, among them the Association for Quality and Participation and the Association for Training and Development. It is the basis of a national award established by Congress in 1987, called the Malcolm Baldrige National Quality Award. And, ironically, given my own initial ignorance, it is rapidly entering spheres outside business. My own university was beginning to institute TQM initiatives toward the end of my research, as was the city of Baltimore.[6] Building on initiatives begun by the Bush administration, the Clinton administration has provided a massive impetus toward developing quality programs in all areas (Solomon 1993).[7]

Even the usual frequent changes in the titles of management programs for the sake of novelty do not seem to be changing the basic content of TQM. The most recent change reported in the business literature is "reengineering"; doubtless there will be others. "Reengineering," at least, does not repudiate TQM, seeking rather more radical means to many of the same ends (Byrne 1993; Hammer and Champy 1993:49).

Most TQM advocates are the belatedly acknowledged heirs of an American statistician, W. Edwards Deming, who played a key role in the reorganization of Japanese industry after World War II. Deming traveled to Japan, studied the Japanese culture and language, and in 1950 convinced the leaders of Japanese industry to adopt his methods stressing quality control and the consumer as the most important part of the production line. Meanwhile, back in America, his ideas fell on deaf ears. Only in 1980, faced with the ascendancy in world markets of Japanese products (owing largely to Deming's method), did the business community in the United States begin to listen to him (Walton 1986:12–14, 17).

Deming's key ideas are that limits of variation of productivity are determined by the system, not by the individual. Hence, quotas, individual measures of productivity, piece work, are all counterproductive because they increase variation among individuals and increase fear.[8] "The result is a company composed of prima donnas, of sparring fiefdoms. People work for themselves, not the company" (Deming quoted in Walton 1986:91). Instead, the job of leaders is to "shrink the control

Incentives:
pride
vs.
competition

limits, to get less and less variation in a process, or less and less difference between people."[9] This is best accomplished without competition: "Look at Moses. He had no competition. Two hundred years ago
Sebastian Bach was writing the rules of harmony for all time. Why did
he do it: Pride of workmanship" (Walton 1986:92, 91).

I entered this terrain of business management as I grew interested
in how health concerns are being handled in U.S. workplaces. Karen-
Sue Taussig and I learned of a new kind of experiential training method
for TQM in which workers and management would climb sheer walls
and tall, slender poles, cross high wires, and jump off cliffs on zip
wires.[10] We were invited to attend a day-long experience run by the
training company Vesta (a fictitious name) for the employees of the
Rockford Company (also fictitious), a multinational corporation in the
top ten of the Fortune 500. Twenty-two thousand Rockford employees were in the process of going through three days of workshops as
well as high and low ropes courses at a rural site on a large bay on the
East Coast.

Protected by sophisticated mountain-climbing ropes and harnesses,
teams of men and women workers and managers of all ages and
physiques (as well as Karen-Sue and I) climbed forty-foot towers and
leaped off into space on a zip line, climbed forty-foot high walls and
rappelled down again, climbed a twenty-five-foot high telephone pole,
which wobbled, stood up on a twelve-inch platform at the top, which
swiveled, turned around 180 degrees, and again leaped off into space.
(This last is privately called the "pamper pole" by the experiential
learning staff because people so often defecate in their pants while trying to stand up on it.)

According to the corporation, this was called "empowered learning."
It is necessary because, according to a Rockford Company brochure,
"We are facing an unprecedented challenge. The world is changing
faster than ever before. Our markets are becoming more complex; our
products are changing; and we are facing global competition on a scale
never before imagined." The brochure continues, "Our survival in the
90's depends upon our ability to change our ways of doing things."
Success in the 1990s, "going over the wall," will require "letting go of
old patterns and behaviors . . . taking a leap through difficult transitions and working hard at new beginnings," "looking forward to change
as a challenge, taking risks and innovating." Emphasis is on a qualitative
break with the way one was in the past; like a caterpillar that transforms
into a different kind of being, a butterfly, people are to be transformed.

The bodily experiences of fear and excitement deliberately aroused on the zip line and the pole are meant to serve as models for what workers will feel in unpredictable work situations. A participant said, "If we could capture the type of energy we experienced on the tower at work, there'd be no limit to what we could do." We were told that the ropes and walls and poles are also meant to scramble the characteristics usually associated with males and females. Men can feel fear on the high ropes course and thereby learn to express their vulnerability; women can feel brave and thereby learn to see their ability to lead. Men and women can also learn to appreciate these unaccustomed capacities in each other.[11] In fact, in our participation in these events, men, even large, muscular men, quite often gave obvious verbal and emotional evidence that they were terrified of heights and confessed, amid much social support from the group, to this vulnerability afterward. (Talk that we overheard among the men about having to go clean out their pants was only barely joking.) Women sometimes also showed their fear and confessed it, but they would receive much more praise from trainers and group members for stoicism, bravery, and physical exertion. In addition to gender barriers, the events are also meant to break down hierarchical barriers between management and labor. Groups that go through the exercises together are usually composed of both management and labor, and a boss might well be depending on his secretary or an assembly line worker to belay him with a rope when he jumps off a tower, and vice versa.[12]

As a participant in the high ropes course, the experience seemed to me emblematic of the kind of spectacular shift in what it means to be a person that has been a theme throughout this book. Although some of the towers that support the activity were made of huge, solidly constructed frames, some of the apparatus was deliberately left loose and wobbly. Many exercises involved walking across a high wire. Not only did I experience the fear of no visible support at a great height, but, on those wobbly poles, wires, or platforms, the fear of being unmoored in space was almost intolerable. The exercises combined the vertigo of standing on the edge of a high cliff with the stomach-dropping feeling of the edge of the cliff itself beginning to crumble. I was literally moving from one position of instability to another and experienced the necessity for great flexibility.

In this terrified condition, each of us was to jump off into space, only to be caught by our harness (belayed by a coworker). There we were allowed to hang (very comfortably, I can report) for a little while,

swinging gently not too far from the ground. The harness completely
and securely supported one's whole torso so that one's reaction was to
slump like a baby in a backpack. As other people jumped before me
and relaxed into this passive, inert posture, I wondered why they did
that. After seeing a photograph of myself hanging in the harness, I realized that I had done exactly the same thing (see fig. 33).

The experience models physically the nature of the new workers
that corporations desire: individuals — men and women — able to risk
the unknown and tolerate fear, willing to explore unknown territories,
but simultaneously able to accept their dependence on the help and
support of their coworkers. In a word, *flexibility*. The isomorphism
between the bodily experience of this training and the results desired
is entirely deliberate: as trainers would often say, we were there to
"experience the metaphor."

An executive of the Rockford Company was very aware of the magnitude of the change that his employees were being asked to make.
Evoking some of the qualities of the passive body and machine-like
work organization familiar from our earlier discussion of the 1940s and
1950s in a speech at a TQM conference, he said, "We made people the
way they are! We can't just throw them away like old, worn-out machinery!! . . . We have treated people in the industrial environment as if
they had no brain. Now they are becoming whole people, and that is
rewarding." These new "whole people" are to be active in their willingness to tolerate risk and danger but passive in their willingness to
depend on the work group. Like the shifting poles, platforms, ropes,
and wires unmoored in space, the nature of the person itself is to shift
and to be able to tolerate continuing shifts.

When I was participating in these events, I had little idea at first
whether they would shed any light at all on other parts of my research
concerning the immune system. I had explained my research to the
executives and trainers as an ethnographic study of concepts of health
and the body in a scientific lab and urban neighborhoods — without
mentioning the immune system specifically. I practically fainted with
astonishment when I discovered that trainers elect to use the image of
the immune system to convey the kind of flexible, innovative change
they desire. While visiting the headquarters of Vesta in the Southwest,
I talked with Mark Sandler, the head of the company and the person
who develops Vesta's training materials. At the end of a long interview,
he asked me to tell him more about my research interests, so I told him
about my research in an immunology lab. He exclaimed, "That is the

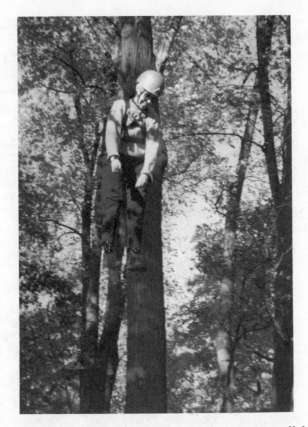

Fig. 33. *Emily Martin hanging in a harness after jumping off the "pamper pole" during a course in experiential training for a corporation.*

very image I use because it works so perfectly to communicate what we want." What he meant to communicate was the image of a flexible and innovative body poised to respond in a continuously changing environment while constantly communicating with other such bodies. Sandler enlisted my help in sending him more material about the immune system that he could incorporate into his training materials: he wanted particularly apt and up-to-date scientific descriptions of how the immune system works.[13]

Later, I realized that Sandler's interest in the immune system was more than metaphoric. At a Vesta workshop on using experiential learning in corporate settings,[14] there was a discussion of psychoneuroimmunology over dinner. It was claimed that experiential learning, which the workshop facilitator referred to as "adrenalin learning,"

immune system

would not only increase the flow of hormones to the brain, thereby increasing learning, but also, through linkages between neuropeptides and the immune system, would improve the health of workers in general. At the level of imagery, and at the level of the physical and mental effects of imagery, trainers at Vesta are deliberately attempting to tap into the interrelated complex systems of the body to produce the kind of workers corporations desire. I took this to be more evidence of the widespread proclivity to think of the body — individual or corporate — as a complex (immune) system.

There is no simple way to pin down how the changes being unleashed by experiential training will work. Marion Taylor, a woman who works at the Rockford Company's technical lab, talked with us throughout the day as we went through the ropes course. She was clearly skeptical about the Vesta experience and referred to it as "brainwashing." In the recent past, she had been active in an attempt (which failed) to organize a union at the company. She told us about many of her complaints at work: sex discrimination, violations of environmental codes, exploitation, and intimidation in general. But, when we visited her several months later at her house near the plant, her understanding of the complexity of the process had changed. In the meantime, a worker had been killed in an industrial accident that many workers believed could have been prevented had management insisted on better maintenance and safety procedures. Marion told us that she now thought Vesta's training had been a good thing: "We got to know each other across divisions there. We never would have trusted each other enough to talk about what happened . . . or to explain our point of view to management."

During my visit to Vesta, one of the trainers told me that I would learn a lot about the implications of these methods from scholars who write about the history and philosophy of experiential learning. Later, I visited some of these scholars in the Midwest, and they were concerned to correct my misperceptions of the scope of experiential learning, misperceptions gained because I had come to know about it through Vesta. They generally considered experiential learning programs for corporations to be marginal, watered down, and designed to sell easily to businessmen for profit. The real heart of experiential learning had a history linked to the development of Outward Bound. Outward Bound began in Wales in 1941 out of a collaboration between an educator, Kurt Hahn, who had opened a school for boys in England, and Lawrence Holt, partner in a British merchant shipping firm. The goal of the educational experience that they provided was "less a train-ing *for* the sea than *through* the sea . . . training through the body, not of the body." Using expeditions on sea and land, they intended to produce "an intense experience surmounting challenges in a natural setting, through which the individual builds his sense of self-worth, the group comes to a heightened awareness of human interdependence, and all grow in concern for those in danger and in need" (Miner 1990:59, 60).

After the war, offshoots of this movement went in several directions. In addition to schools in the United States and England modeled directly on Outward Bound (Greene and Thompson 1990; Loynes 1990), academic departments focused on experiential learning were founded in two places. One of the two Coors Beer brothers endowed the department at the University of Colorado, and Dewitt Wallace, the owner/editor of the *Reader's Digest*, endowed the department at Mankato, Minnesota. Both departments grant master's degrees in experiential education and run experiential learning programs on high and low ropes courses for local community and school groups.[15]

Experiential educators believe that the techniques of experiential education provide a key to opening individuals and groups to higher moral and ethical states of being and a greater degree of self-actual-ization in all areas of living. One team of psychologists singles out expe-riential education as likely to increase the experience of "flow" in all areas of life (Csikszentmihalyi and Csikszentmihalyi 1990:154). With this emphasis, they place themselves within a tradition of thinking and practice that is long-established and runs deep in American culture, that of self-help and improvement. One contemporary example of this pull-oneself-up-by-the-bootstrap tradition was often cited to me as essential reading and referred to in the lectures, seminars, and con-ventions that I attended on workplace training.

This is a book called *Developing a 21st Century Mind* by Marsha Sinetar. A key part of a twenty-first-century mind is "creative adapta-tion," which "generates personal reinvention and develops inner bal-ance, self-trust, experimentation, and the blossoming of intuitive intel-ligence. It implies continual, appropriate adjustment to a changing field of opportunities — not a onetime response to a single disruption (Sinetar 1991:12). In the book, Sinetar describes a client who was "rigid and unbending and . . . could not 'go with the flow.'" . . . "Her goal was to become more flexible and innovative (both qualities exist within the synergy of the creative adaptive skills complex)" (p. 37). To increase her flexibility, Sinetar recommended that the client practice writing

with her left hand and, following this, take up interpretive dance
(p. 13). For Sinetar, dance is not just a metaphor for the desired ability — flexibility. It is therapy: "George Leonard writes that primitive
dance can be viewed as a metaphor for life itself. . . . The more deeply
we see into life, the more clearly we perceive the dance. Pursuing reality down into the heart of the atom, we find nothing at all except
vibration, music, dancing" (p. 82).

It is startling how often the image of the dance is used to capture
the nonhierarchical character of groups made up of individuals who
creatively adapt, constantly adjusting to changes in the environment
and each other. Recall the ads for Nike shoes, the tango of the
designer-architect-builder, the dance of the stretching, flexible body,
Kantor's "giant with the agility of a dancer," the "skinless man" posed
like a dancer on the cover of *Science*, and Bateson's balancing acrobat.
The dance is also frequently used as an image to capture the nonhierarchical nature of a complex system of entities that are constantly
adjusting to each other. Recall the "intricate dance" of the cells of the
immune system, Bubbles the B cell "dancing about," and the image of
immune cells as Fred Astaire dancing with Ginger Rogers. The qualities associated with dance — flexibility, grace, balance, mutual interaction, delicate adjustment — make it an image that can capture the
qualities now required of good workers (as well as healthy bodies). As
figures 34 and 35 demonstrate, even computer engineers can dance
the maypole with their printouts; even stagehands dance a ballet with
their props and controls.

In a less benign image than the dance, however, much of the self-
help literature on work and experiential training urges people to tolerate serious, life-threatening risks, whether in the constructed environment of experiential learning or in the precarious job market. Some
authors advocate actually seeking out life-threatening risk. Arguing for
"rescue-free" wilderness areas, designated places where no state-
funded rescue is permitted, McAvoy explains that a "general insurance
mentality" in American society makes these areas desirable: "Many
people want to be protected from all risk. They want the benefits of
high-adventure activities (personal growth, stimulation, enhanced
awareness, self-fulfillment), but they want the potential costs to be
borne by others, usually the government. . . . Persons with this insurance mentality want illusions of challenge, risk, and self-reliance, but
they want a government-sponsored safety net" (1990:331).

In developing a philosophical justification of the value of danger and risk, Jasper Hunt draws on Plato: "From Plato the argument is put forth that no, all danger should not be avoided; the use of danger is justified by making better people; and care must be taken to rescue the young people if too much danger presents itself" (Hunt 1990:123). Hunt continues, quoting with approval from a lecture by the modern adventure educator and philosopher William Unsoeld:

> I've got to put in a pitch for risk. Because somehow, I see our youth of today being conditioned in the other side of the tracks too much, being warped over here to the conviction that, if it's *risky* it's *bad*. I think that you pay too great a price when you excise risk from your total economy. We used to tell them in Outward Bound, when a parent would come and ask us, "Can you *guarantee* the safety of our son, Johnny?" And we finally decided to meet it head-on. We would say, "No. We certainly can't Ma'am. We guarantee you the genuine chance of his death. And if we could guarantee his safety, the program would not be worth running. We do make one guarantee, as one parent to another. If you succeed in protecting your boy, as you are doing now, and as it's your motherly duty to do, you know, we applaud your watch dog tenacity. You should be protecting him. But, if you succeed, *we guarantee you the death of his soul!*"

Two trainers at Vesta explained to us how risk and fear are managed on the ropes course:

> MATT SANFORD: Height is one way. I'm finding it a very universal fear factor. I like to say, as I've heard it said before, everyone's afraid of heights. It just happens at different heights. You know? I mean, you get somebody who's not afraid to stand up on top of a thirty-foot pole, you put him on top of a 225-foot skyscraper standing at the end looking off, and I bet they're a little bit nervous about something.
> SANDRA SALZBERG: A perfect example is, I do all the events all the time, and when we were in Spain, we climbed up these stairs in a cathedral with no hand railings, this spiral staircase, you're probably four hundred feet up, and I had to go down, and it was like, OK, I've had enough, I'm going down now.

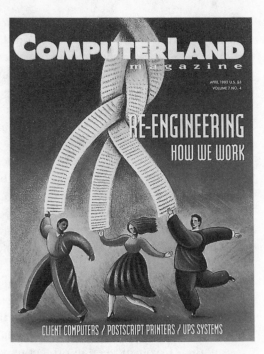

Fig. 34. *How computer engineers dance the maypole. From the cover of* Computerland, *April 1992.*

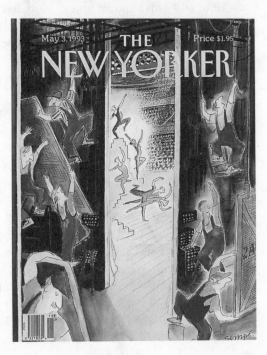

Fig. 35. *"Ballet's new spring," showing how stagehands dance as they work backstage, just as the dancers do onstage. From the* New Yorker, *3 May 1993. Cover drawing by Sempé; © 1993 The New Yorker Magazine, Inc.*

MS: So it's one way to get a person in a stressful situation, see what that brings up, to compare that to a stressful situation, how they reacted there compared to how they react in a stressful situation in the workplace, being one of the main reasons. Another being, why are you afraid is the big, the kicker. The whole thing for me comes down to perceived risk and actual risk. You think you're going to die, it's a scary thing. You've been assured that you won't, the safety systems are pretty meticulous, and you're ensured of those, and, again, why should I take somebody's word for it, that's a good question to ask. . . . And maybe, then, you just deal with the concepts of perceived and actual risk, which happens in all of our lives. I mean, I can't leave my job even though I'm unhappy because, you know, I'll have no money and I'll lose my house and I'll starve and I'll die. You know? And we can make those scenarios look pretty bad in a hurry, and then reality is, no, I'll have to buckle down a little bit. I'll have to get more creative, find a new job, and in the long run it might be better, you know? And it might be a little risk of, yeah, you might die. But to at least have a handle, it's the easiest way I think to, throughout the spectrum of people we're dealing with, to get them in a situation where there's perceived risk, and it's stressful, and you're among peers. And a lot of times peers, where you don't want them to see that you're afraid, because you work with them and they think you're the rock. And you're five feet off the ground, your secretary just did it.

The owner of another experiential education firm confirms that fear of the unknown is used to intensify stress and speed up learning: the goal is to put a person in "the most unnatural situation that we can very quickly so that learning is dramatic and it's quick. . . . When you get people off the ground, they're scared. It's an unnatural place for humans to be. *We're not squirrels*" (Kimberly Leeman).

Teaching people to tolerate life-threatening risk is hardly an abstract matter. The risks sometimes involve serious and frightening threats. The changes at Rockford Company, for example, are being implemented only after substantial delayering, downsizing, or, in old-fashioned terms, firing a significant portion of the workforce. A film that we were shown at the Rockford plant and a slide presentation put together by the head of Rockford's human resources program that we saw at the corporate headquarters both stressed the drastic reduction of the company's workforce during the 1970s and 1980s. Many of the people "delayered" were in middle management. Most of the literature on training stresses the ubiquity of these processes: downsizing, delayering, the obsolescence of middle management, careers that will be made up of "hopping" from one job to another rather than a continuous trajectory in one company (Kantor 1989; Deal and Kennedy 1982). Clearly, the executive who said, "We can't just throw [people] away like old, worn-out machinery," was being somewhat disingenuous.

Toleration of risk will be demanded from management as well as labor: management must accept a dramatic reduction in its numbers and must expect to grant some form of ownership of the company to its workers. Many experiments with various forms of profit or stock sharing are under way. At the moment, the Rockford Company has discontinued its first experiment, "variable pay," in which a portion of a worker's pay would go up or down with the company's profits, and begun a second experimental stock option plan.[16]

Not a few of the people we interviewed on the subject of health were undergoing one or another of these "downsizing" processes. They are so common that "unemployment" is sometimes listed as an illness state in material on how the immune system is affected by stress! The study that recommended confession as a way to a healthier immune system found that workers who regularly confessed in writing their deepest feelings about the loss of their jobs found another job faster than those who did not (Dreher 1992:77). Karl Gossner, who until recently had worked for an insurance company, reflected:

> I believe in change. On the other hand, believing in change, I got to be the first person that's going to take the good with the bad, and I kind of have to realize that even in my own life things are going to change a lot. And as a result of this last layoff, I've come to realize that this is probably going to be the way the rest of my life is. Any concept I had, like go into a company and stay there, work, work my way through it, around it, up and down it for the next twenty or thirty years, that's just not realistic. . . . The more I talk to my friends who are in diverse businesses, engineers, and just other fields, it seems that it's happening to everybody. There's a lot more turnover in the careers — [if] a lot of things are now going on in a project, a lot of staffing goes in, in these little binges.

Staff up for a project, and then, if things slow down, you unstaff for it.

There seems to be a wide consensus that the best way to cope with "unstaffing" is to increase one's education. In his election campaign, Clinton "redefined job security." He said repeatedly that the middle classes would have to undergo lifetime training and reeducation, be prepared to change jobs and even careers regularly (Neikirk 1992). Statements about the necessity of continuous education have been common, but they are getting stronger of late. Peter Drucker recently claimed that, what the feudal knight was to the early Middle Ages and what the bourgeois was to capitalism, the educated person will be "in the post-capitalist society in which knowledge has become the central resource" (1993:211). W. Edwards Deming claims that "profound knowledge" will be required for individuals to "reenforce each other for accomplishment of the aim of the system" (Deming 1993:94).

Given the positive value accorded education in American culture, pronouncements about the increasing importance of education are usually made in a very optimistic tone, like Drucker's, but sometimes they can be made in a wry tone of futility and despair, as in Garry Trudeau's evocation of the "disposable worker's" hopelessness (see fig. 36). Sometimes the positive challenge of obtaining more education is recommended in a way that makes the reasons for the disposable worker's hopelessness and fear apparent:

> [In "workplace 2000,"] continuous learning will become commonplace to create a more flexible work force, provide employees with the skills necessary to take advantage of rapidly changing technology, and prepare employees for new jobs inside or outside the company when their old jobs are replaced by technology or eliminated due to changes in customer demands. To be successful, Americans will have to seek out training opportunities to supplement their existing skills and to learn new skills. (Boyett and Conn 1991:7–8)

Human resource managers see themselves as midwives helping old, stiff, rigid organizations die and new, flexible, innovative ones be born. They describe themselves as agents of change who lead individuals on journeys during which their old selves die to give birth to new persons,

persons who take risks, innovate, flexibly adapt to constant change, supercharge their immune systems, and work effectively in complex groups for the good of the whole corporation, persons who, all the while, glance uneasily over a terrifying edge into an abyss, inhabited by the unemployed, underemployed, temporarily employed, and destitute, fearing extinction from neglect and disease.

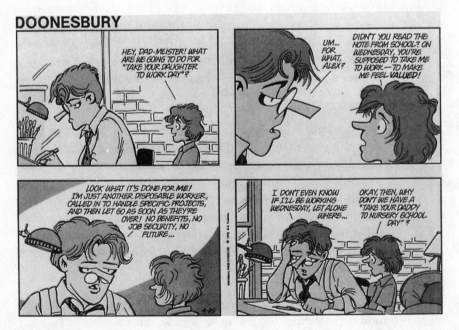

Fig. 36. *Retraining the disposable worker.*
"*Doonesbury*" © 1993 G.B. Trudeau. *Reprinted with permission of Universal Press Syndicate. All rights reserved.*

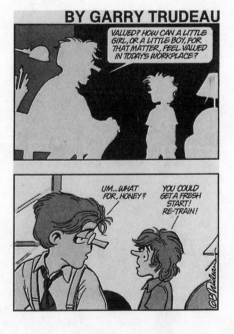

PART
SIX

POST-DARWINISM

There were perhaps two thousand Indians living on Cape Cod when the Pilgrims arrived. No one knew for certain. But white diseases had already begun their work on the naive immune systems of the native American. Within a century and a half, there were only five hundred adult Indians on Cape Cod. Their ancestors had sold most of their lands for kettles and English hoes, then moved to reservations, known as plantations, or to Praying Towns where well-meaning ministers taught of the white god who sent diseases in his wrath and took them away in his mercy.

WILLIAM MARTIN, *Cape Cod*

Is the immune system at the heart of a new incarnation of social Darwinism that allows people of different "quality" to be distinguished from each other?[1] I believe that the answer may be yes, and, in this final chapter, I want to identify some of the strands of this disturbing development.

These days, we are often warned that an apocalypse of disease is coming soon, in which all of us will be tested but only some of us will survive.[2] Oddly enough, most of these warnings do not involve AIDS. The writer Richard Goldstein points out (Goldstein 1991) that, until very recently, mass media coverage of AIDS positioned the general reader or viewer as a witness to HIV, but a witness who is safely immune to it. Since Goldstein wrote, there has been a move afoot in the popular press to reposition the general public in such a way that the general public "we" is depicted as just as much at risk from disastrous epidemics as the special populations who were once depicted as the only people threatened by AIDS. The position of "the public" has moved from safe witness to participant in impending disaster.

For example, Richard Preston's 1992 *New Yorker* article, "Crisis in the Hot Zone," contains horrifying descriptions of the effects of Ebola virus: "You can't fight [it] off . . . the way you fight off a cold. Ebola seems to crush the immune system. The virus perhaps makes immuno-suppressant proteins . . . which — if, indeed, they exist — would act as molecular bombs that ruin parts of the immune system, enabling the virus to multiply without opposition." Ebola causes the body to melt, liquefy, so that the slimes and uncoagulated blood that run from the cadaver are saturated with Ebola virus particles: "That may be one of Ebola's strategies for success: the melting body oozes Ebola virus across body boundaries to other hosts." But, beyond graphic description, the key argument of the article is this:

> The emergence of [viruses like Ebola and] AIDS appears to be a natural consequence of the ruin of the tropical biosphere. Unknown viruses are coming out of the equatorial wildernesses of the earth and discovering the human race. It seems to be happening as a result of the destruction of tropical habitats. You might call AIDS the revenge of the rain forest. . . . Some of the people who worry in a professional capacity about viruses have begun to wonder whether H.I.V. isn't the only rain forest virus that will sweep the world. The human immunodeficiency virus looks like an example rather than a culminating disaster. As lethal viruses go, H.I.V. is by no means nature's preeminent display of power. The rain forest, being by far the earth's largest reservoir of both plant and animal species, is also its largest reservoir of viruses, since all living things carry viruses. . . . When an ecosystem suffers degradation, many species die out and a few survivor species have population explosions. Viruses in a damaged ecosystem can come under extreme selective pressure. Viruses are adaptable: they react to change and can mutate fast, and they can jump among species of hosts. As people enter the forest and clear it, viruses come out, carried in their survivor-hosts — rodents, insects, soft ticks — and the viruses meet *Homo sapiens*. (Preston 1992:59, 62)

This passage evokes the horror of a system gone out of control that we have seen is so prevalent in current cultural images of disease. Destruction of the rain forest ecosystem allows viruses to escape control and explode, mutating quickly and jumping species. Ebola transmits itself by contact with the liquefying corpse; as the borders of the body are destroyed, the virus leaks into the world to wreak destruction elsewhere.

The inescapability of contemporary epidemics was emphasized as well in the *New York Times Magazine*, in the guise of an article on the flu (Henig 1992). This article places AIDS in the context of the numbers of people who died in previous flu epidemics: in 1918, influenza killed 196,000 people in this country during the single month of

October, more than twice as many as died of AIDS during the first ten years of that epidemic. By the end of 1918, between 20 and 40 million worldwide had died. Not only, the article implies, is AIDS not much by comparison with this record of fatalities, but it is not much by comparison with the super abilities of the flu virus: whereas HIV (a lentivirus) evolves slowly (although it mutates rapidly inside its host), the influenza virus has "mastered . . . just one terrific trick: the speed with which it evolves" (p. 30). This means that those of us who contract the flu in one year "will have little immunological memory for the slightly changed virus a year later" (p. 64). It is not clear just whose immune system will be able to survive the threat of the next "major plague" (p. 67) caused by the flu, whose toll will be, finally(?), appalling.

These articles accomplish two significant things. First, the public is drawn to participate in the horror of possibly succumbing to a deadly epidemic, but this is done at the cost of displacing attention away from HIV/AIDS and onto hypothetical, and presumably far worse, diseases. Second, there is an apocalyptic tone to the writing, a sense that the world as we have known it is going to come to an end in some disaster wrought by microbes.[3] But, even in the midst of evoking disaster, there is more than a hint that *some* people with the right kind of immune systems will survive.

Something of what it is to have the *right* kind of immune system is made clear in an article called "The Arrow of Disease" (Diamond 1992) in the magazine *Discover*. Diamond poses the question: "When Columbus and his successors invaded the Americas, the most potent weapon they carried was their germs. But why didn't deadly disease flow in the other direction, from the New World to the Old?" (p. 64).

Before answering this question, the article explains that the oldest diseases of humanity are characteristic of small, isolated populations. Crowd diseases appeared with buildup of large, dense human populations. The rise of agriculture, the rise of cities, the development of world trade routes, all this meant a field day for crowd diseases. In these circumstances, the source of new diseases was often animals and pets.

With the *European* invasion of America, "far more Native Americans died in bed than on the battlefield — the victims of germs, not of guns and swords. . . . The main killers were European germs, to which the Indians had never been exposed and against which they therefore had neither immunologic nor genetic resistance. Smallpox, measles, influenza, and typhus competed for top rank among the killers. As if those were not enough, pertussis, plague, tuberculosis, diphtheria, mumps, malaria, and yellow fever came close behind" (Diamond 1992:72). The reader is given the clear impression that the Native Americans must never have been exposed to crowd diseases such as smallpox, measles, influenza, and typhus. Only after this does the author note there were populous towns and cities in both North and South America and that the total population was comparable to Europe.

The conclusion is that, even though the Native Americans had "crowds," they may have started their population rise later than Europe (and so had less time to evolve); their three population centers were not connected by regular, fast trade "into one gigantic breeding ground for microbes, in the way that Europe, North Africa, India, and China became connected in the late Roman times" (Diamond 1992:73); and they did not have as many domesticated animals. So it was the Europeans' more potent germs that made the conquests possible. The not quite hidden subtext is that the Europeans' immune systems had evolved to a higher state as a result of being challenged by more evolved, newer, and nastier germs.

The logic behind the argument in this article is one example of cultural processes by which new versions of old hierarchies are being put forth, hierarchies in which some of us have fit enough immune systems to survive plagues and some of us are fated to succumb. It is also a way to reveal processes by which our attention is diverted from AIDS and HIV, a current plague that it is no exaggeration to call horrible.[4]

Popular writing about emerging new viruses and the differentially fit immune systems of "peoples" of the Old and New Worlds is very theoretical. A much more concrete and grounded representation of differential survival occurred in the integrated community of Warren, with its high levels of unemployment and poverty. John Marcellino, the community leader we met discussing electron micrographs, spoke of the community's poor health, malformed bodies, and general neglect:

> Or, like, I got bad teeth, OK? And one of the things all poor people have is bad teeth, because of being poor, OK? . . . It's one of the first things I noticed when I started moving around, because, when I talk to Indian people, they got bad teeth. You know what I mean? And I go down South, and they got bad

teeth, so it's one of the things that poor people share all over
the world in common. We all got bad teeth. You know what I
mean? [Laughs.] And what I come to realize it's for a number
of reasons. One is, I think that government doesn't want us to
have, they don't care about our teeth. . . . I never could figure it
out. It just pissed me off, you know what I mean, but I figure
it's one of the ways of distinguishing poor people from the rest
of the population is we all got bad teeth. [Laughs.] . . . And so
you won't get rid of the drug abuse or the prostitution or the
crime or stuff until the people who live here are no longer here.
And that to me is the same as the underclass thing, *disposable*
people. . . . As soon as they can't figure out a need for us, they'll
get rid of us.

What's the need for you right now?

We still make money for somebody or another. They still need
us some, like they needed people to come up out of the South
to work in the mills, so they attract them all up. Now there's not
as much need for the people to work in the mills, they need
some people in the service economy, they try to retrain . . . but
if not they're no use, they'll put you in jail. . . . They'll choke
you off so that you can't make a living doing anything else, so
they get rid of you, or, you know, hopefully you'll go back to
Virginia or somewhere else, right? You know, you'll crawl in a
crack, or you won't have children, or something.

Neither the bodies nor the communities that Marcellino is describing
are likely to be able to adapt successfully to serious challenges:

We think it [AIDS] could kill us. It could just kill a lot of people
in our community, that's what I think about. Because, with
AIDS, the way they say that you get AIDS, we got a lot of relationships here, because they say that you get AIDS through
needles, and a lot of our people shoot up. They say you get
AIDS through gay sex, and a lot of our people function as pros-
titutes, and are [a] really sexually active population, so, and
then you get it through having relations with one another, and
you pass it by being close to one another, and our people are
very close to one another.

Close?

You know what I mean . . . like the way to not get AIDS is to not touch people, you know what I mean? That was the way it first came to us. You know, and then as we learn more and more about it, you know, we learn that it's real specific in terms of how you can catch it. You know like being monogamous and only having one partner, you know what I mean, and that kind of stuff. That's not usual in our community, particularly among young people and, you know what I mean. But it's not usual, and then you have all this interaction between needle users and folks involved in prostitution, and a lot of interaction in the community, and so it's not like separated, it's not like, well there's a needle community up here, and people shoot up, and they don't have nothing to do with our community. They're part of our community, and having relations in our community, and there's people who, you know, are involved in male prostitution, you know what I mean? And they're over here, you know, and there's a gay community over there, you know. It's integrated in our community. So our fear was, oh my God, you know, when I first heard about it, I thought, Jesus, we're going to be like death.

When was this?

This was maybe seven years ago or so. It was before people were even talking much about it. We just heard, and I thought, Jesus, if they say that you get it in these two ways, and there's a lot of that in our community, gee, we're going to, you know, this is horrible. And I went to the hospital, you know?

To get tested?

No, I went to the hospital to say you got to do something. You know what I mean? I went, this is God's honest truth, I went up to the hospital there, it was called Public Health Hospital, and I said we need to know more about this stuff because this stuff's going to kill us. It's going to wipe us out. You know, and I was sure we were going to have an epidemic because if what they were telling us was true, we would. What I know is when I looked into it, we haven't had nobody dead.

Really?

Nobody. And I don't understand why. . . . Then they said, OK, and this is a real glitch, because then they said it can be seven years before you know you have it, and I thought, well Jesus

Christ then, we're really in trouble. 'Cause now, all these people got it, but nobody knows they got it, right? And eventually
it's going to be like, you know, all of a sudden it's going to be
like, you know, like a butterfly, you know? [It's a] little thing,
and all of a sudden . . . one day it's all going to be, you know, all
through the community.

John Marcellino fears the loss of the life of an entire community, a
"little thing" like a caterpillar that will grow into a big thing like a butterfly, signifying not rebirth but death "all through the community."[5]
As we have seen, elsewhere in the social hierarchy, in the training
grounds of major corporations, people are using the image of caterpillars and butterflies in a starkly different way. In these corporations
(speaking only of those who survive "delayering"), "mechanical" workers will be reborn to a new life as "flexible" workers; caterpillars will be
reborn as butterflies.

As MARCELLINO'S comments about teeth suggest, health can operate as
a single standard of comparison among people or among groups of people. In our interviews, there were many instances in which people used
the immune system this way. People made comparisons between individuals: "Some people have stronger immune systems than others, just
because of the way they're made up" (Gillian Lewis); you get HIV
while another person does not because "maybe your immune system
just isn't as beefed up" (John Parker). People also made comparisons
between groups: women don't get AIDS as much as men because they
have stronger immune systems (Carol Neilson); people without a good
living standard need vaccines, whereas vaccines would only clog up the
more refined immune systems of middle-class or upper-class people
(Barry Folsom).

The mechanism by which the immune systems of people and
groups are seen to vary, when people explained it, is invariably a version
of Darwin's notion of survival of the fittest:

If you have the master key to all the doors on this floor, it's possible that there will be one door that, say the lock is old or the lock
is new or something, and the master key will not fit that lock, and
therefore you cannot get into that room. And so, you-we would
say that room is resistant to that key or that lock is resistant to the

key, and so, even if you tried a million times, you still couldn't get
that key in there. . . . There's this notion that the host, since we're
all slightly different in some way or another, they actually say if
you want to think about it, a lock and key analogy, they don't have
the right lock. These things that cause disease like viruses and
every other thing, they're tricky. They have evolved to recognize
our locks. And so every once in a while they're going to encounter
a lock that they've never seen before because either that person
is evolutionarily behind the times or they're evolutionarily ahead
of the times. So that's how I would explain how some people don't
get disease. (Bruce Kleiner)

As another scientist explained, "There are legitimately immune systems
that are more powerful than other immune systems" (Peter Keller).
The struggle goes on for some at every level, from cells to living organisms:

You know how like life is a struggle from the smallest bacterial
critter all the way up to lions and tigers and bears and everybody's
kind of struggling to survive. Well, you can actually take that sort
of like even smaller down to the cell level, like cells trying to hang
on. For example, when your whole body is out in the cold freez-
ing, your body sort of just says, Well, let's sacrifice the fingers. So
you actually cut the blood off to your fingers and . . . you just try
to spare the core so you can sort of just look at that like as long
as everybody's happy, everybody's happy. Decisions get made.
The weakest and least important get sacrificed. (Hal Packard)

A scale measuring people and groups in terms of their immune
strength allows some people to feel especially potent. Not a few people
we interviewed, especially young male doctors or medical students,
expressed a kind of immune machismo. One medical resident I heard
about, dismissing the possibility of contracting HIV infection from
blood in the emergency room where he worked, claimed that his
immune system could "kick ass" (George Stocking, personal communication). And, in an invidious twist, the local newspaper reported that
"5 Texas girls say they had sex with an HIV-infected male to get into
gang": "If the test came up negative, then it was like they were brave to
have unprotected sex and they were tough enough and their body was
tough enough to fight the disease" ("Five Texas Girls" 1993:7).

These sorts of evaluations emerge very readily in our interviews from the logic of the immune system as a currency of health; they can also be found throughout the popular literature on health:[6] "We are not all born equal when it comes to the T cell system. . . . The consequences of having a second-class T cell system are enormous" (Dwyer 1988:44). People vary in "the quality of their immune systems" (Edidin 1991:49). Sometimes these evaluations fit easily over older hierarchies: in a radio report on the different susceptibilities of people to valley fever in southwest California, we learn that "dark-skinned people — Latinos, Filipinos, and African-Americans — are more at risk for serious forms of the disease. Researchers' theory to explain this is that "people respond differently depending on their genetics; but as the immune response differs according to the genetic material that you have . . . that determines how well or how poorly you do when you get infected by certain agents" ("Morning Edition," National Public Radio, 5 January 1993).

Although Dwyer, Edidin, and NPR are referring to the effect of genetic variability on the immune system, texts equally often mention the effect of what kind of "training" we give our immune systems: "Like an army which is prepared and waiting but never called into action, an unused immune system may become obsolete, not sufficiently prepared for new types of attack" (Pearsall 1987:39).

The notion that, through practice and training, one can develop an immune system more able to survive threats introduces a mechanism of survival very different from the genetic givens that operate in natural selection. One of our immuno-macho doctors had his immune system in a training program:

> Like, for example, eating things that are not particularly well cleaned, or, you know, go on trips and drink water from a river, and, it's sort of, to build up my immune system. Now, I don't know if it has any advantage for me, or if actually I'm exposing myself to any more danger, and I guess I should think a little bit more about that, but that's sort of my little idiosyncratic attitude about my own immune system. I'm trying to train it, sometimes.
> *To train it?*
> Yeah. [Laughs.]
> *Do you like to challenge it, or what?*
> Yeah, yeah. (Ken Holden)

The notion of training the immune system can also be found in parts of new age thought, in which the immune system, interlocked with other bodily systems, is treated as the key to the evolution of higher states of being.[7] The most fully developed example of this genre of which I know is Michael Murphy's encyclopedic, *The Future of the Body* (1992). In Murphy's design, the complexly interrelated systems within the body, to which the immune system is central, are the grounds on which the possibility of imminent evolution of the human species to a "higher level" is based:

> The findings of psychoneuroimmunology and related fields reveal: (1) the highly interactive, feedback-laced nature of psychophysical functioning; (2) multiple ways in which particular alterations of consciousness, behavior, bodily structure and process are mediated; and (3) the immense specificity with which significant changes are happening, moment by moment, throughout the nervous, endocrine, and immune systems. A body so mutable and interactive, operating with such redundancy and specificity, seems more capable of the transformations described in this book than a tightly compartmentalized, poorly articulated organism would be. (p. 23)

Murphy envisions the development of "extraordinary functioning," which heralds the coming of a new "evolutionary transcendence," involving a "new level of existence that has begun to appear on earth" (pp. 25–27). "A break with ordinary human activity" would constitute a "new kind of life on this planet" (p. 28). The manifestation of this "greater life . . . latent in the human race" (p. 30) will be an evolutionary jump on the same order as the beginning of life itself and the origin of *Homo sapiens*.

While it is not clear from Murphy's account *who* will be capable of this evolutionary jump, it is clear that the training to make it possible is elaborate. The second half of the nearly eight-hundred-page book is a handbook of techniques and practices that might help: yoga, Rolfing, meditation, breathing exercises, and the martial arts, to name only a few. Many of us, from medical doctors to anthropologists (including this anthropologist), no doubt follow more than one of these practices and find them rewarding and health enchancing. But it does not require much extrapolation to raise the question of how *limited* access to the kind of intense evolutionary training that Murphy advocates may be. Training of the elaborate sort that Murphy outlines takes money, time, information, and opportunity, things in short supply for many people, including those in the community described by John Marcellino.[8]

The strands that I have been tracing here evoke some very old linkages between biological and social realms. They are reminiscent of some of the ways in which social value systems were rooted in biological theories in the nineteenth century.[9] But there are important ways in which today's "survival-of-the-fittest" visions differ from those of the nineteenth century.[10] Writing about the forms that racism is taking in Europe at the end of the twentieth century, Etienne Balibar begins by marking the distance between racism today and racism in the recent past:

> It [racism today] is a racism whose dominant theme is not biological heredity but the insurmountability of cultural differences, a racism which, at first sight, does not postulate the superiority of certain groups or peoples in relation to others but "only" the harmfulness of abolishing frontiers, the incompatibility of life-styles and traditions; in short, it is what P. A. Taguieff has rightly called a *differentialist racism*. . . . It is granted from the outset that races do not constitute isolable biological units and that in reality there are no "human races." (1991a:21)

But, even though the terms have changed, Balibar argues, the processes inherent in racism — "the categorization of humanity into artificially isolated types" (1991b:9), the "need to purify the social body, to preserve 'one's own' or 'our' identity from all forms of mixing, interbreeding or invasion," and to articulate this around "'stigmata of otherness' which might be name, skin color or religious practice" (1991a:17, 18) — have very much continued.[11] What has happened is that *culture* now takes the place once occupied by biology, to lock individuals and groups "a priori into a genealogy, into a determination that is immutable and intangible in origin" (p. 22). In sum, "culture can also function like a nature" (1991a:22).[12]

In another account of new forms of racism in Europe, Verena Stolcke distinguishes what she calls "cultural fundamentalism" from an older racism: "Cultural fundamentalism purports to justify the exclusion of *foreigners, strangers* thought to threaten national cum cultural identity and unity, [while] racism serves to justify the socio-economic inferiority of the *underprivileged*, be they at home or abroad." Both forms have in common that they conceal specific conflicts of interest under the guise of "natural facts": "This 'naturalization' is predicated on an exaltation of incommensurable difference — of cultures in anti-immigration rhetoric, and of individual 'talents' in that of social inequality" (1992:29).

Balibar's and Stolcke's alertness to new ways of measuring and monitoring people in forms of racism in Europe raises interesting questions about how the immune system might be operating in a ranking of people in the United States. As I said, we often found people willing to make comparative estimates about the quality of different people's immune systems. Although some people probably had comparisons based on genetic substances in mind, some were thinking along the very different lines of evolution through training. The notion of training contains as its first premise that people can change their behavior and attitudes if they are exposed to the right environment. The notion of mind and body inextricably enmeshed in a complexly interacting system means that any change in behavior or attitude will affect one's health and, unavoidably, one's immune system. Some people have taken up a notion of adaptation that is, like training, based on practice and potentially available to anyone. Unlike Darwinism, the outcome is not linked to the original biological material with which one was born. This kind of evolutionary adaptation is focused on the ever-changing individual in his or her unique environment.

It is clear to me that what is at stake in our understanding of "health" are the broadest issues of the survival and death of the social order itself. In the workplace settings that I have already described, we came across an elaborate theory of evolution by training that sheds light on how we know who will survive. The two human resource managers Cary Nelson and Lauren Gershon, for example, told us that the object of their training programs is to develop a higher-order organization: "If you have two halves that are whole and you put them together, you come up with a third whole, which is greater than those two other wholes. When you have two halves, you have just that, two halves, two incompletes. We want a whole people functioning as a whole unit . . . this great ring of wholeness." In developing their policies, they "look at things from a systems model." They recommended a book called *The Paradigm Shift* in which the author shows how, if the system shifts, we then shift in our part of the system. They told us that this shifting process resembles Rupert Sheldrake's theory of "morphic resonance": "The way it works is if we are trained . . . if we get enough people to do this [any action], this becomes available to the mass sub-conscious." Morphic resonance is also known as "the hundredth mon-key" theory, they explained to us:[13]

> Ninety-nine monkeys learned the process of washing a piece of fruit or a banana on an island. When the hundredth monkey in that pack learned that behavior, on another island a hundred miles away, that group of monkeys started that same behavior [the first] hundred over here had learned. That's called the morphogenetic resonance field. [The first] group of monkeys set up that pattern for that other group of monkeys to pick up.
> *Across space?*
> Yeah. Across time-space barriers.
> *And what is the name of the consciousness?*
> Group subconsciousness.

We have no way of knowing how widespread acquaintance with Sheldrake's ideas is among people we interviewed. After Cary Nelson and Lauren Gershon spelled the theory out so clearly, we realized that several other people had been implicitly using his ideas without our realizing it. It is worth noting that his books are widely available in paperback editions (Sheldrake 1988, 1991). His ideas have also been widely disseminated in the press: in 1993, for example, his theories were discussed in fifty-three newspapers nationally as well as in *Time*, *Newsweek*, *Esquire*, and *Science Digest*.

I cannot do justice to the complexity of Sheldrake's ideas here or to their potential for providing a critique of establishment science. At the least, however, it is clear that Sheldrake's ideas provided Cary Nelson and Lauren Gershon a metaphoric, if not a literal, way of understand-ing how a change in one part of a complex system can jump in a non-linear way across time-space barriers to effect a change in another part. This was meaningful to them in their effort to lead their organization into a higher-order state, a state in which it might stand a chance of surviving in the harsh environment it faced.

In the overall realm of opinions we heard expressed about how in the near future some organizations and people will survive and some perish, Sheldrake's ideas were hardly the most curious, at least to a novice, such as I am, in the intricacies of new age thought. During an interview with Rebecca Petrides, an authority on new age matters, I wondered aloud why the concept of the immune system has been adopted so quickly by the general public. I asked her whether she thought one reason might be because the immune system resonates with much older concepts of health, such as humoral models of the body. She responded with enthusiasm, making plain the millennial aspect that she believed was important in the present era: "You're probably right, and I think that, when you look at the way information comes through a society, there is such a thing as consciousness, you know, that hundredth monkey theory. And I think that's at play now in all these things, when you have sort of like [what] the Hindus call . . . the end of the dark age. And in other esoteric systems, this is really the end of a very big, 25,000-year cycle, which is why it's so cataclysmic and so difficult."

Commenting that she wanted to "throw something in just for the fun of it," Rebecca told us that another piece of the coming cataclysm has to do with people who have been abducted as part of an extraterrestrial breeding program. Potential participants in the program are put through "tests" — for example, their "shakras are measured" — and then alien fetuses may be implanted in them. The reason for this program is that "some of the alien civilizations, their bodies are weakening. Their immune systems are weakening from being in space so long that now they need to interbreed. And so there are interbreeding programs that are going on, and that's been pretty well documented, it's just a question of when will the public be told this has been going on."

Since I did not specifically seek out practitioners of new age thought during my research, my knowledge of the ways in which its various versions elaborate differential survival at the millennium is very limited. Still, I am struck that at least some strains of new age thought stress how differential survival can be determined by training.

In this way, new age thought shares something with the many people who probably knew nothing about Sheldrake's or other new age theories, who used education and training as the determinant of evolutionary survival. Bruce Kleiner guessed that the level of AIDS would level off in the United States but go on to become catastrophic in Africa and other Third World countries. In this country during the polio epidemics of the 1940s and 1950s, we "got used to" avoiding infectious people. The germ theory has been "pounded into our heads." "It's very easy for us to wrap our minds around the notion of AIDS as an infectious disease as a contagious thing" because of the "general level of education." "We're on the far side of the jungle floor."

"Our conception of immunology is much more sophisticated and allows us here in this country to take the necessary means. . . . We have no problem understanding what disease is about." Because they lack these forms of training and education, African societies will not be able to survive: "That notion of a virus itself is alien to a Ugandan tribesman. And asking him to wear a condom is like asking him to wear a trash can over his head when he goes to see his favorite girl. What are you wearing a trash can for? . . . So that's why I think it's going to be a big problem."

This concept of earnable competence, hinging on a core notion of trainability and educability, powerfully reflects the peculiarly American cultural attachment to individual growth and development, as expressed from Horatio Alger to Bill Clinton. The heights of achievement are open to all who will work hard and apply self-discipline. In an article entitled "A Brave New Darwinian Workplace," *Fortune* spells out the problem: as rigidly hierarchical schemes for organizing work are destroyed, schemes that have limited the ability of "people, organizations and markets to behave in *natural ways*," the transition will "be brutal for all concerned, but . . . the workplace will be healthier, saner, more creative, and yet more chaotic — *like nature itself.*" The necessary realization then becomes to "forget old notions of advancement and loyalty. In a more flexible, more chaotic world of work you're responsible for your career. For the adaptable, it's a good deal." The solution is that "specialization is out, a new-style generalism is in. The most employable people will be flexible folk who can move easily from one function to another, integrating diverse disciplines and perspectives" (Sherman 1993:51, 50, 52; emphasis added). In a sense, "training" becomes "natural" here, much as Balibar argued "culture" could become. And, like the "nature" of anything, this different basis for inequality does seems *not arbitrary or artificial* to us but rather based on good sense, progress, or the fruits of knowledge.

There are also, however, some fundamental differences between a "nature" of race or culture and a "natural" selection based on a *training* model. In Balibar's terms, race and culture operate within and between social *groups*, by means of artificially isolated types, a purified social body, identities preserved from mixing, and a stigma of otherness. In contrast, training — of the immune system, the body, the self, or the soul — can be a *solitary* matter. There is no end to ways in which each person can privately follow programs, regimes, and self-help plans (like those in Murphy's book), some even complete with tests to monitor your progress. One self-help way to assess your own immune system's functioning is the "Immune Power Final Exam" in *Fighting Disease* (Michaud and Feinstein 1989:371–72). You get a high score if you "walk at least three times a week," "act like an optimist, even when you feel like a grump," "know how many lymphocytes you have on the job," and "do a good deed every day" (p. 372).

Race and culture are grounded in communities, as John Marcellino saw only too well: it was the "integration" of the community that was to be its downfall under the threat of HIV. But the operations of training seem to be unmoored from place. As Lauren and Cary put it, this kind of learning works "across time-space barriers." In a sense, the whole story of the hundredth monkey is a parable that says that spatial separation (or proximity) *does not matter*.[14] Making spatial relations irrelevant can cause the very particular face-to-face relationships produced in communities and workplaces to seem to disappear. If morphic resonance allows you to link up with others who, like you, have been exposed to advanced training, you can ignore those down on the ground and in between who, perhaps because they have been "unstaffed," could not participate.

The idea of morphic resonance operating across time-space barriers may also appeal to the dramatically altered experience that we have of time and space in the era of flexible specialization. Time-space compression affects us all, as our work lives are sped up and electronic communication links us instantaneously around the globe. But some of us, with access to E-mail, fax machines, computers, and jet travel, can orbit in hyperspace, while some of us will still be stuck on the ground. Financier Jacques Attali describes the characteristics of the emerging "empowered, liberated nomads." This nomadic elite "is already forming, severing its ties with any particular place, whether nation or neighborhood" (1991:88).

The form that training is taking in the workplace today, as we have seen, positively seeks hybrid groups, mixing genders and gender roles, diverse ethnic backgrounds, and so on. What Cary Nelson called the "ring of wholeness" binds management and labor, supplier and manufacturer, manufacturer and customer, into wholly unaccustomed, startling new relationships on a global scale. In trying to trace the outlines of the selves and bodies populating this scene, the stakes are very large. At stake is what kinds of bodies we imagine will be able to survive the next eruption of Ebola or the development of a more virulent flu or crowd disease. At stake is what kind of mechanism we imagine will enable some of us — and not others — to evolve into successful, healthy workers, surviving in higher-order organizations.

Survival is a key term here because it entails a notion of comparative vitality: the extinction of some is constituted by the witnessing of the survivors:

> What prompts survival concerns is not simply the vision of an imminent exit from the sensuous, future-binding life, saturated with hope and expectation, but the awareness that others will go on living. . . . Survival concerns always include, therefore, the comparative aspect: immortality not being a viable option, survival means living *longer than others*. Though born of the ostensibly universal human condition, survival concerns differentiate. . . . Those about to survive me will be spectators of the impending revelation of my nothingness. It is their gaze that will constitute my nothingness. (Bauman 1992b:26)

AT THE BEGINNING of my research, I wondered whether it would be possible to understand how the economic and social formation of late capitalism can influence "culture," in particular, internal and external forms of the body in health and illness. Certainly, others have argued that aspects of late capitalism are responsible for the form taken by such cultural productions as architecture, art, or literature (Jameson 1984; Harvey 1989).[15] Now that my research has been concluded, it seems to me that, when it comes to the disciplines of science and medicine, given their cultural preeminence in the United States, one could as feasibly argue that the ideal models of being in the world that these disciplines generate (i.e., the innovative, agile body) could be acting as templates for ideal forms of conducting business or making products (the innovative, agile firm).[16] That is why I adopted the tactic of moving back and forth between descriptions of "cultural" and "political economic" realms, allowing them, for the interim, to have putative autonomy. Knowing that I was unable to determine the precise causal nature of their connection (if, indeed, there is any), I simply wanted to raise the question: What new images and forms of the body and kinds of powers that regulate it are coming into existence contemporaneously with the dramatic shift in political economic organization that is being brought about by flexible specialization?

At the beginning of my research, I also wondered whether "scientific" information just traveled out of the lab into the culture and there had its effects, period. As the research went along, I learned how often, as in the case of electron micrographs, the effects of scientific information could lack altogether the kind of closure that could be produced inside the lab. Consequently, it seemed possible that there would be many roads by which the kinds of cultural understandings of the body and health that I have described throughout this book could return to transform knowledge within the laboratory itself. It is perhaps too much to expect to catch this process "in the act"; the process is likely to be ineffable, made up of implicit understandings and preoccupations that permeate the ideas and practices of scientists in daily life, as in their work.

Despite the difficulty of *proving* the existence of this process, however, there are many suggestive indications that it occurs:

- We have traced in detail the emergence of an "unnerving new view of man's place in the world" (Alpers 1983:17) taking place in many arenas involving a variety of forms of systems thinking. Is it unreasonable to think that this new view might have played a part in the shift within science — still under way — to seeing the body as defended by a complex internal *system* in the first place?
- My immunologist colleague Mike Edidin chose the image of an ancient fortress, a monumental edifice defended with moats and walls against a hostile enemy, to describe the immune system; Vera Michaels chose the image of "waves," evoking a turbulent, chaotic, complex phenomenon, in constant change. Edidin's image stresses stable, secure *defense*; Michaels's stresses a complex, turbulent *system*. As models in the science of immunology shift away from the defended castle to that of the part embedded in a complex whole, giving up the strict self-nonself distinction, will this development not likely be partially influenced by a cultural environment in which this shift of body image has *already taken place* in many areas outside science and in the private musings of many scientists as well? In this case, immunology is having a path beaten to its door.
- The nearly universal understanding of health in any of its aspects in terms of the immune system, a process that is fueled

by the findings of scientific research on the immune system as translated by the media, surely must influence the thinking of the politicians who approve financial allocations, the scientists who approve research grant applications, the scientists and editors who select what papers get published, and so on. Finding out more about how the immune system works or what it influences is understood as a viable and productive activity. Freud used the notion of "overdetermination" to describe a phenomenon with many causes, none sufficient in itself, but together more than sufficient.[17] To stay with the imagery of roads and paths, we might say that a ten-lane superhighway would barely be sufficient to handle the ideas and practices treating the body, self, and world as complex systems that must be shuttling back and forth between the general culture and the scientific community involved in research on the immune system.

What is most troubling to me about the new cultural sensibilities that I have been describing is the very thoroughness with which (immune) systems thinking has permeated our culture. I find this development troubling because, for all the beguiling attractions of this way of positioning oneself in the world, it also has disturbing implications. There is the propensity to extol harmony within the system and reliance on the group while paradoxically (and distractingly) allotting individuals a dynamic, ever-changing, flexible role. As we saw earlier, concealing conflict between those who have different amounts of resources and power for the sake of the appearance of harmony usually hurts the disadvantaged. There is a propensity to imagine systems as inexorably evolving wholes while simultaneously setting up comparisons with other systems that cannot survive. As we saw earlier, this propensity plays its part in an emerging form of neo–social Darwinism, which again has unfortunate consequences for the disadvantaged.

Perhaps the seductiveness of (immune) systems thinking comes about because it seems to represent an escape from earlier forms of discipline that constrained bodies and groups in the mass production era, the strict immobilization of the body in rigid postures and limited movements in factories and prisons or the detailed rules that governed mind and body in schools and the military (see Foucault 1979, 1980).[18] Fresh from these experiences, it is no wonder that moving gracefully as an agile, dancing, flexible worker/person/body feels like a liberation, even if one is moving across a tightrope. But can we simultaneously realize that the new flexible bodies are also highly constrained? They cannot stop moving, they cannot grow stiff and rigid, or they will fall off the "tightrope" of life and die. We need to examine carefully the social consequences of these constraints.

I began with Norma Field's (1991) poignant description of the repressiveness of everyday life in Japan. Her narrative counteracts this repressiveness by describing people in Japan who have managed to resist the national harmony that is enjoined, refusing to forget the past, sometimes at great personal cost. During our fieldwork, we often met people who are resisting models of the body (as a machine), or of vaccines (as beneficial state education), or of work (as a hierarchical bureaucracy). But the models that they are resisting are already in the process of transformation. In their resistance, these people often embrace a vigorously emerging systems thinking that may embody entirely new forms of repression.[19] In many ways, we are all being enmeshed by the alluring web of systems thinking. My hope is that, with eyes a little more open, we might realize one thing: although we now think of ourselves and our world as complex systems, we have not always seen things this way. We have changed our views of the world in the past, and it is very possible that we will want to change them again.

At the moment, many (myself included) may feel delight at some of the changes being brought about in the new flexible corporations: the elimination of some old hierarchies between management and labor, the effort to include women and minorities, the integration of mental and manual skills on the job, the wish to treat workers as whole people. Equally appealing may be the ideal person who will hold jobs in these corporations: a lean, agile, innovative, flexible soul, who will be whole in mind and body and will nimbly manage a multitude of life relationships and circumstances to maintain a vigorous state of health. The trouble is that this ideal (as would any) rests on a *narrow* vision of the able person, one that will discriminate against many people. Keeping this in mind might allow us to broaden our notion of who is fit to survive in this world. Even as economic processes may seem to force our *corporations* to become flexible, lean, and agile, perhaps when it comes to *persons* we could relish both the flexible, lean, and agile and the stable, ample, and still.

Even as corporations downsize, unstaff, and delayer, we need deliberately to keep in mind the physical and emotional effects of these processes on the delayered workers in near or distant communities.

Even as we may be caught up in the seductive appeal of jobs that entail flexibility — home working, telecommuting, multitasking — we need to remember the cost, which may include loss of pensions, health insurance, and unemployment insurance.[20] In the face of the incitement to be nimble and in constant motion, we need to remember the common human need for stability, security, and stasis. The challenge is to sustain our critical perceptions in a culture that prizes being flexibly adaptive without allowing our perceptions to become so flexibly adaptive that they can only compliantly perpetuate — instead of calling attention to — the order of things.

ALTHOUGH this is the final section of the final part, I have carefully avoided labeling it *conclusion*. A more accurate label would be *on the impossibility of concluding*. In part, it is impossible to conclude because the book consists of observations about processes that are still in process. The molten nature of the contexts that I have described and their relations with each other would make it foolhardy for me to predict the shape that all this will take in the future.

In part, it is impossible to conclude because there is no vantage point from which I can say confidently that the developments that I have described are "good" or "bad." Or, rather, there is no *one* vantage point but instead a very great *many* vantage points from which such evaluations can be made. In a sense, the structure of the book itself, tracking its way from one vantage point to another but making none of them the foundation, is an index of this feature of the world we are making.

The structure of the book is also an index of the extent to which people in a great many walks of life participate in making the world-view that is currently emerging. No matter how massive and overwhelming the process of world concept formation feels, so all pervasive as it is, it is important to remember that almost all of us have participated in making this happen. We are not victims of a sinister plot perpetuated by villainous others but active participants in a complex process. I intentionally designed the book around the words and experiences of a large number of people in order to make visible the existence of this widespread participation. And of course such widespread participation meant that, from the start, unless our research embraced people from all walks of life, we would never be able to make sense of what was happening.

I completely understand (indeed feel myself) the desire for *closure* at this point. What has caused all this? What will happen next? Is it a good thing or a bad? But the desire for a single perspective that would make sense of it all must be inevitably frustrated. This is so not only because we are still living through what we would like to encompass and completely understand but also because the prospect of a single explanation is itself rendered impossible by the processes through which we are living. The development of the complex systems model that seems so salient to us in so many contexts, the model that seems to underlie the organization of our bodies, our groups, our work settings, our world — this model itself repudiates any notion of a structure built on one foundation, an explanation that rests on one principle. In turn, the complexly interconnected world in which we now live seems to say that both the model and its implications fit the current nature of reality. All is in flux, order is transient, nothing is independent, everything relates to everything else, and no one subsystem is ever necessarily continuously in charge.

The findings in this book were constituted by the insights of many people, and therein lies one solution to the dilemma of what the reader is to do with the disquiet that may be left by its disturbing revelations. What is needed, as systems thinking develops in further directions as yet unknown, is for everyone who is willing to attend to the configurations and practicums falling into place around us — at work, school, home, clinic, or hospital — to notice these things and to think critically about them. This would form a continuing harvest from the acute attentiveness and critical sensibility to our culture and society so evident in the words of the many people who speak in this book.

APPENDIX 1

The Neighborhoods

In spite of the occupational and spatial shifts that many people have experienced in the last two decades, Baltimore residents continue by and large to see themselves as belonging to particular geographic neighborhoods, each with a distinct set of historical and socioeconomic characteristics. Below, I sketch each of the main neighborhoods in which we focused our fieldwork, in the words of their residents. (To preserve anonymity, I have not made detailed reference here to published histories of Baltimore neighborhoods. Some of those available are Waesche [1987], Fee, Shopes, and Zeidman [1991], and Olson [1980].)

STOCKTON is a neighborhood of mostly white working-class families, who live in the neat two-story brick row houses, each with a small yard in front and another in back. A minister in the neighborhood comments on its insularity and consequent reputation for racial intolerance:

> This is a community that has been virtually all white forever, and it's also a community that has a certain amount of Klan presence and activity. And I think also it's a community that considers itself somewhat beleaguered, I suppose. The housing opportunities are really getting more and more scarce for the people here, and I think it's pretty scary to think about what's going to happen as rents keep going up, and people's incomes don't, and there's not enough. There's just not enough, and if this becomes a place where rents are lowest in the city, we have to share them with everybody, there's not going to be enough for us. (Joe Elliott)

251

Our research in Stockton led us to other neighborhoods just over its borders. The first of these, MONTCLAIR, is home to primarily African-American working-class people who live in small row houses much like those in Stockton. Whereas in past generations many Stockton residents worked in the textile mills on the nearby river, people in Montclair worked for white people in the wealthy neighborhood of Hamilton on the other side of them from Stockton: "[Montclair residents] didn't work in the mill. They worked in service and what not. Chauffeurs, cooks, and gardeners and things like that. That's the first generation. Then the second generation started bringing teachers, doctors, lawyers, and things like that" (Mildred Cosgrove). Today, residents delight in the neighborhood's safe, clean, and "respectable" nature: "People mind their own business, and, well, like Friday night, Saturday night is just like Sunday morning, they're all quiet, and all nice days and nights. . . . People of all ages, and it's a wonderful place to rear your children. Very nice. It's safe" (Fran Diamond).

The wealthy community of HAMILTON, with large single-family houses on spacious, landscaped lots is concerned with its borders and its integrity, as Stockton is. A resident explains:

> Well, the primary issues we're concerned with relate to maintaining the integrity of the area. . . . There are covenants on most of the properties in Hamilton, which means that the owners cannot do whatever they want with the property, but they have to relate to certain standards that we try to maintain, so that the neighborhood doesn't deteriorate or become nonrecognizable. . . . There's a procedure that you have to go through to make changes to your property, and that's related to the covenants, which are actually part of the deed of the house and are passed on from owner to owner, from generation to generation. . . . So when I say *integrity* I mean to maintain the residential characteristics of Hamilton. (Russell Lambert)

On the edge of Stockton, facing a swath of green fields and trees, is the somewhat more upscale community of RIVERDALE. A resident of Riverdale who moved there from Stockton compares the two:

How is Riverdale different from Stockton?
Well, having my porch canvassed with Ku Klux Klan flyers, for

one thing, was disturbing, although there's a contingent in the neighborhood which was also trying to get a neighborhood association going against specific groups which discriminated against people, which was good. . . . People take a long time to accept you in that neighborhood, and they're not very open. And when they see you are a student, they don't really know what to expect. And so I think it's sort of nerve racking for them. . . . Our neighbors, you know, on this side are really wonderful to us. They've helped us out, helped us fix things in the house. . . . We know most everybody in the whole block. There's a mixture. There's young people, people with families, but then some older people too. And they're mostly professional people. I mean it does make a difference if you feel more comfortable with people who are like you. (Rachel Cole)

Around the other side of Stockton from Riverdale is WARREN, a chronically poor, integrated neighborhood, plagued with high unemployment. One resident describes it as "regular working folk, but there's some poor sections. . . . We're like a poor suburb of Stockton. . . . Folks are poorer, folks are a lot more victim of circumstance down here. . . . The majority of the people were born and raised here. . . . There's been more history with integration here than there has in Stockton, where there's been no history, or [a] bad history" (John Marcellino).

On the other side of the city, some distance from Stockton and its surrounding neighborhoods, is FRANKLIN. Made up of narrow single-family or attached houses, the neighborhood lines up for several blocks on either side of a busy but rundown street of shops and offices. Unlike any of the neighborhoods described so far, nearly everyone singles out diversity as its hallmark: "There's that real sense of community. It's diverse that there are a lot of blacks and whites, a lot of young students, a significant number of retired people, and a lot of people raising families, so that there's quite a few children around. Makes for what I think [is] a very nice group. There's a little bit of tension, racial tension I think. I think it's probably less than most communities, but it is there" (David Feldman). There is also class tension, as some people are "struggling just to eat, . . . just to keep ahead, you know, just to keep their homes together" (Bonnie Germano), while others are concerned about increasing the value of their property:

If my adjacent neighbor lets his roof deteriorate to the point where it leaks, the water then gets into my house and starts to deteriorate my house. So everybody who has adjoining houses has to understand that, not only are they sacrificing their own property, but they're impinging on the people adjacent to them. If I'm not a basically fairly sanitary person, I'll have roaches. Well, everybody knows that in the city, if one house has roaches, then the next three have roaches, so, and rats. If you don't keep your yard cleaned up, you'll have rats, and so will your neighbors. (Bill Slocum)

South of both Stockton and Franklin, and more or less equidistant from both of them, is MONTGOMERY. The area is a conglomerate of tall apartment buildings, stately nineteenth-century town houses, and streets of shops, restaurants, and businesses ranging from the elegant to the funky. Like Franklin, it is economically diverse, but within greater extreme limits: "There's really no way to pigeonhole the neighborhood at all. I mean, just in my one block, you know, from the rental, you know, the apartment building that's right next door to me that has six apartments, to the house across the street that is a grand Victorian house and would probably sell for about $175,000. Just the extremes, just within my one little block, are immense. So it's tough to generalize" (Mary Loran). Like Franklin, Montgomery is also socially diverse, including the strong presence of the gay and lesbian community as well as its community organization headquarters: "The demographics in Montgomery break down roughly to about 30, 35 percent senior citizens, about 40 or 45 percent gay and lesbian, about, and the remaining factor is mostly young, heterosexual, professional couples, students, again a lot of people in the other two groups fall into the students and then professional scene as well, you know, that type of thing. It's a neat area because it is so diverse" (Charles Kingsley).

APPENDIX 2

The People We Interviewed

Only people with whom we held sustained, relatively systematic tape-recorded conversations are listed here. Overall, we interviewed 225 people: 49 percent women and 51 percent men; 73 percent Euro-American, 26 percent African-American, and 1 percent Asian-American. (According to the U.S. Census of 1990, out of the 2,382,172 people who live in the Baltimore metropolitan area, 71.7 percent are white, 25.9 percent are black, 1.8 percent are Asian, and 0.3 percent are Native American [Clayton and Campbell 1992:36]). Of the people we interviewed, 30 percent were forty or older, 44 percent were younger than thirty, and 25 percent were in their thirties. The median age in Baltimore is 33.4 years (Clayton and Campbell 1992:36). For those we interviewed through the ALIVE (AIDS Link to Intravenous Experiences) study, we were sometimes not able to get complete biographical information because of their difficult life circumstances. Only people we interviewed in connection with their residence in a Baltimore neighborhood have a neighborhood listed after their names. People we met in other contexts — alternative health clinics, HIV/AIDS organizations, immunology classes or laboratories, corporations, experiential education organizations, etc. — do not have their residence listed.

Able, Elizabeth, F, 20s, Euro-American, college senior
Abrahams, Becky, F, 20s, Euro-American, immunology graduate student
Alvin, Mike, M, 20s, African-American, biology research scientist
Aronson, Teri, F, 20s, Euro-American, immunology graduate student

Baltzer, Linda, F, 50s, Euro-American, Stockton, live-in companion
Bannister, Ralph, M, 30s, Euro-American, Warren, financial reporter
Becker, Vivian, F, 40s, Euro-American, immunology professor
Black, Peter, M, 20s, Montgomery, Euro-American, waiter
Blackstone, Mary, F, 40s, African-American, Franklin, unemployed
Blackwell, Jim, M, 30s, African-American, ALIVE
Blanchard, John, M, 30s, Euro-American, environmental protection
    organization employee
Bonnell, Arnold, M, 20s, Euro-American, Riverdale, insurance salesperson
Booth, Eleanor, F, 60s, Euro-American, Stockton, retired nurse
Borel, Shelley, F, 20s, African-American, immunology graduate student
Boswell, Peter, M, 40s, Euro-American, M.D.
Bowler, Edith, F, 70s, Euro-American, Stockton, retired
Bowler, Victor, M, 70s, Euro-American, Stockton, retired mill worker
Braun, John, M, 70s, Euro-American, Montgomery, retired
Breslau, Joan, F, 20s, Euro-American, Franklin, translator
Browner, Allan, M, 40s, Euro-American, homeopathic M.D.
Chappell, Ron, M, 30s, Euro-American, Montgomery, therapist
Chase, Allan, M, 20s, Euro-American, medical student
Christopher, Sarah, F, 20s, African-American, Montgomery, fast-food
    restaurant worker
Cole, Rachel, F, 20s, Euro-American, Riverdale, public health graduate
    student
Cooper, Dawn, F, 18+, African-American, Franklin
Cosgrove, Mildred, F, 60s, African-American, Montclair, retired
Cosgrove, William, M, 60s, African-American, Montclair, retired and part-
    time worker in an electronics factory
Coulter, Erwin, M, 30s, African-American, ALIVE
Cowan, Paulette, F, 18+, African-American, Franklin
Crofton, Daniel, M, 40s, Euro-American, Hamilton, data processor
Currant, Jimmy, M, 30s, African-American, ALIVE
Daniel, Teresa, F, 18+, African-American, Franklin
Davies, Robert, M, 30s, Euro-American, M.D.
Demarco, Lisa, F, 20s, Euro-American, Franklin, HIV/AIDS service
    organization counselor
Diamond, Fran, F, 60s, African-American, Montclair, retired
Drucker, Bill, M, 30s, Euro-American, retail shop manager
Early, Brian, M, 30s, Euro-American, technician in immunology lab
Egloff, Jane, F, 20s, Euro-American, secretary and AIDS activist
Elliott, Joe, M, 40s, Euro-American, Stockton, minister
Fanzini, Mike, M, 20s, Euro-American, college senior
Feldman, David, M, 20s, Euro-American, Franklin, graduate student
Felton, Sally, F, 20s, Euro-American, Franklin, secretary

Fetzer, Jenny, F, 30s, Euro-American, Franklin, HIV/AIDS social worker

Fisher, Sabine, F, 20s, Euro-American, masseuse

Folsom, Barry, M, 40s, Euro-American, acupuncturist, herbalist

Forbes, Dena, F, 40s, Euro-American, epidemiologist

Fordham, Carina, F, African-American, ALIVE

Franklin, Jewell, F, 30s, Euro-American, Montgomery, special education teacher

Franz, Gladys, F, 70s, Euro-American, Stockton, retired

Franz, Herman, M, 70s, Euro-American, Stockton, retired autoworker

Franzini, Mike, M, 20s, Euro-American, college senior

Gaspari, Sarah, F, 20s, Euro-American, immunology graduate student

Germane, Ned, M, 20s, Euro-American, Franklin, HIV/AIDS service organization employee

Germano, Bonnie, F, 30s, Euro-American, Franklin, computer operator

Gershon, Laura, F, 40s, Euro-American, human resources director

Godwin, Sue, F, 30s, Euro-American, social worker in HIV/AIDS counseling

Gonzalez, Laura, F, 20s, Euro-American, Franklin, unemployed

Goodale, Hariett, F, 30s, Euro-American, biological research technician

Gorden, Ray, M, African-American, ALIVE

Gossner, Karl, M, 30s, Euro-American, laid off from insurance industry

Green, Eliot, M, 30s, Euro-American, Franklin, architect

Gregory, Robert, M, African-American, ALIVE

Greiber, Martin, M, 20s, Euro-American, immunology graduate student

Hale, Beth, F, 20s, African-American, Franklin

Harrison, Arthur, M, 20s, Euro-American, musician

Hayes, Janice, F, 40s, Euro-American, retail salesperson

Hedley, Derek, M, African-American, ALIVE

Henry, Bryan, M, 50s, Euro-American, ROTC faculty member

Hensler, Sid, M, 30s, Euro-American, ROTC faculty member

Higden, Anita, F, 30s, Euro-American, owner of hair salon

Hill, Sheree, F, 20s, African-American, Franklin, unemployed

Holcolm, Tara, F, 20, African-American, Franklin, unemployed

Holden, Ken, M, 30s, Euro-American, molecular biology postdoctoral fellow

Houlihan, Elizabeth, F, 20s, Euro-American, Montgomery, teacher

Huff, Daryl, M, 20s, Euro-American, Montgomery, salesman

Humphreys, Anthony, M, 30s, Euro-American, acupuncturist

Hunter, Aaron, M, 50s, Euro-American, immunologist

Jackson, Donald, M, African-American, ALIVE

Jenkins, Steve, M, African-American, ALIVE

Jester, Steve, M, 20, Euro-American, technician in immunology lab

Johnson, Katherine, F, 30s, Euro-American, Franklin, midwife

Johnston, Earl, M, African-American, ALIVE

Jones, Gladys, F, 30s, African-American, ALIVE

Kahn, Zena, F, 30s, Euro-American, Franklin, nursing student

Kantor, Sam, M, African-American, ALIVE

Kelder, Valerie, F, 30s, African-American, Franklin, computers

Keller, Peter, M, 40s, Euro-American, biology professor

Kelsey, Charlene, F, 20s, Euro-American, Montgomery, police officer

Kessler, Cindy, F, 40s, African-American, Franklin, AIDS hotline worker

Ketcham, Sherry, F, 40s, Euro-American, works for Vesta, experiential
   education for corporations

Kingsley, Charles, M, 30s, Euro-American, Montgomery, insurance
   company employee

Kleiner, Bruce, M, Euro-American, M.D., research associate in biology

Knight, Duane, M, African-American, ALIVE

Kohler, Eva, F, 20s, African-American, Montgomery, hotel worker

Kohtua, Don, M, 20s, Asian-American, retail manager

Ladlaw, Cindy, F, 30s, Euro-American, Franklin, photographer

Lambert, Russell, M, 50s, Euro-American, Hamilton, M.D. and professor

Lamont, Franklin, M, 20s, African-American, custodian

Landers, Marcia, F, 20s, Euro-American, federal AIDS/HIV researcher

Langford, Michael, M, African-American, ALIVE

Larson, Cynthia, F, 40s, Euro-American, M.D.

Lavinson, Jeff, M, 20s, Euro-American, federal education policy adviser

Leeman, Kimberly, F, 30s, Euro-American, president of experiential
   education organization

Lennox, Cary, F, 20s, Euro-American, college sophomore

Lerchen, Guy, M, 20s, Euro-American, M.D./Ph.D. student

Lewis, Gillian, F, 20s, Euro-American, Montgomery, librarian

Lockard, Judy, F, 40s, Euro-American, Hamilton, federal employee

Loran, Mary, F, 30s, Euro-American, Montgomery, real estate agent

Lyon, Sandra, F, African-American, ALIVE

McCarty, Diedre, F, 50s, Euro-American, Stockton, administrative director

McClain, Jeff, M, 30s, Euro-American, Riverdale, lawyer

McGuire, Barbara, F, 40s, Euro-American, Montgomery, attorney's
   employee

McKenna, Cindy, F, 20s, Euro-American, HIV/AIDS service organization
   worker

Makefield, Sharon, F, 70s, Euro-American, Stockton, retired

Mandell, Rose, F, 20s, African-American, Franklin, unemployed

Marano, John, M, 30s, Euro-American, Stockton, M.D.

Marano, Judy, F, 30s, Euro-American, Stockton, teacher

Marcellino, John, M, 40s, Euro-American, Warren, community organizer

Marey, Abby, F, 20s, Euro-American, Montgomery, investment bank
   employee

Marshak, Dan, M, 20s, Euro-American, biology research technician
Marshall, Wendy, F, 40s, Euro-American, Franklin, social worker
Marson, Jack, M, 70s, Euro-American, Franklin, retired seaman
Mattson, Stephen, M, 20s, Euro-American, Montgomery, teacher
Maxwell, Teresa, F, 20s, African-American, Franklin, shelter worker
Mayfield, Julia, F, 60s, Euro-American, Hamilton, retired
Michaels, Vera, F, 30s, Euro-American, Stockton, lawyer
Miller, George, M, 20s, Euro-American, Montgomery, insurance company
    employee
Millner, Hugh, M, 40s, Euro-American, holistic M.D.
Miner, Horace, M, African-American, ALIVE
Monroe, Phillip, M, 20s, Euro-American, Montgomery, accountant
Moore, Nancy, F, 40s, Euro-American, Franklin, nurse
Morgan, Jack, M, 70s, Euro-American, retired seaman
Morris, Sol, M, 40s, Euro-American, Stockton, funeral director
Neilson, Carol, F, 30s, Euro-American, Montgomery, bartender
Nelson, Cary, M, 30s, African-American, human resource office employee
Norton, Jack, M, 20s, Euro-American, HIV/AIDS service organization
    employee
Novick, Martha, F, 20s, Euro-American, college sophomore
O'Grady, Michael, M, 40s, Euro-American, immunology professor
O'Hara, Patricia, F, 40s, Euro-American, acupuncturist
Olson, Fred, M, 40s, Euro-American, immunology professor
Oreck, David, M, 30s, Euro-American, M.D. researcher/professor
Owen, Briwn, M, African-American, ALIVE
Packard, Hal, M, 20s, Euro-American, postdoctoral biology student
Parker, John, M, 20s, Euro-American, Montgomery, financial adviser
Perkins, Mary, F, 30s, Euro-American, homemaker
Peters, Goeff, M, 30s, Euro-American, Montgomery, graduate student
Peterson, Laura, F, 30s, Euro-American, Stockton, nurse
Petrides, Rebecca, F, 40s, Euro-American, director of holistic health center
Pierman, Marve, F, 30s, Euro-American, Riverdale, social security employee
Pirone, Cathy, F, 40s, Euro-American, laboratory technician and biology
    graduate student
Pitasky, Anne, F, 20s, Euro-American, immunology graduate student
Pittman, Robyn, F, 50s, Euro-American, Riverdale, geologist
Porter, William, M, African-American, ALIVE
Rabinow, Martin, M, 30s, Euro-American, MD, nutritional M.D.
Radlaw, Cindy, F, 30s, Euro-American, filmmaker
Randall, Becky, F, 40s, Euro-American, Stockton, health administrator
Rangra, Kay, F, 20s, Asian-American, Montgomery, word processor
Ritchie, Lynn, F, 30s, Euro-American, Franklin, dairy worker
Robertson, Joel, M, 20s, Euro-American, Montgomery, reporter

Roche, Carmen, F, 30s, Euro-American, Franklin, teacher

Rockel, Michelle, F, 40s, Euro-American, Stockton, immigration service employee

Rodriguez, Peter, M, 20s, Euro-American, Montgomery, epidemiology graduate student

Romanoff, Jane, F, 40s, Euro-American, psychologist

Rose, Craig, F, 30s, Euro-American, director of Vesta, experiential education for corporations

Rosen, Linda, F, 50s, Euro-American, Stockton, nurse

Ross, Harry, M, 20s, Euro-American, Montgomery, works for HIV/AIDS organizations

Salzberg, Sandra, F, 20s, Euro-American, Vesta employee

Samuels, Beverly, F, 70s, Euro-American, Franklin, retired clerk

Sanborne, Joyce, F, 40s, Euro-American, Riverdale, lawyer

Sandler, Mark, M, 50s, Euro-American, president of Vesta, experiential education for corporations

Sanford, Matt, M, 20s, Euro-American, Vesta employee

Sansom, Lynell, F, 40s, African-American, Stockton, director of shelter

Sargent, James, M, African-American, ALIVE

Sarton, Julia, F, 40s, African-American, Franklin, teacher

Saviano, Frank, M, 40s, Euro-American, nutritionist

Schulman, Philip, M, 40s, Euro-American, Montgomery, social worker

Scofield, Luther, M, African-American, ALIVE

Scott, Mark, M, 30s, Euro-American, designer

Seaman, Leon, M, African-American, ALIVE

Silverstein, Paul, M, 30s, Euro-American, Franklin, employee of publisher

Simpson, Joe, M, 30s, African-American, ALIVE

Sloane, Meredith, F, 30s, Euro-American, humanities professor

Slocum, Bill, M, 20s, Euro-American, Franklin, architect

Smith, Jack, M, 70s, Euro-American, Montgomery, retired

Solomon, Laverne, F, 50s, African-American, foundation employee

Spicer, Michael, M, 20s, Euro-American, Montgomery, psychiatric researcher

Stevens, Frank, M, 30s, African-American, ALIVE

Stokes, Anthony, M, 30s, Euro-American, temporary employment agency staff

Stone, Homer, M, 30s, African-American, ALIVE

Stratton, Drew, F, 20s, Euro-American, college senior

Sullivan, Gary, M, 30s, Euro-American, Hamilton, lawyer

Tanner, Claude, M, 30s, Euro-American, M.D. and professor

Tapper, Gretchen, F, 20s, Euro-American, immunology graduate student

Taylor, Marion, F, 40s, Euro-American, Rockford employee

Thompson, Brackette, F, 18+, African-American, Montclair, high school student

Thompson, Mark, M, 40s, Euro-American, biology professor

Torok, Brian, M, 20s, Euro-American, Montgomery, medical laboratory technician

Torres, Deborah, F, 30s, Euro-American, Montgomery, veterinary employee

Towers, Sophia, F, 20s, Euro-American, accountant

Tracer, Jack, M, 70s, Euro-American, Stockton, retired sheriff

VanHorn, Peter, M, 40s, Euro-American, immunologist

Vanross, Ed, M, 40s, African-American, ALIVE

Wade, Sara, F, 20s, Euro-American, immunization techician

Wagner, Adam, M, 20s, Euro-American, college sophomore

Walden, Chris, F, 30s, Euro-American, biology technician

Walker, Leon, M, 30s, African-American, ALIVE

Wallace, Frank, M, 20s, Euro-American Montgomery, oil company employee

Walter, Tyrone, M, African-American, ALIVE

Walton, Richard, M, 40s, Euro-American, immunology researcher

Weisser, Ernest, M, 40s, Euro-American, experiential education professor

West, Leroy, M, African-American, ALIVE

White, Martin, M, African-American, ALIVE

Whitman, Mara, F, 30s, Euro-American, Montgomery, technical writer

Wilcox, Janey, F, 30s, Euro-American, Montclair, self-employed office manager

Wilder, Ron, M, 30s, Euro-American, M.D.

Wilkenson, Mary, F, 20s, Euro-American, biology graduate student

Williams, Patrick, M, 30s, African-American, artist, ALIVE

Willis, Elva, F, 40s, African-American, Franklin, social worker

Wilmslow, Marsha, F, 20s, Euro-American, Montgomery, medical laboratory technician

Wilson, Harry, M, 40s, Euro-American, Stockton, computers

Wilton, Mary, F, African-American, ALIVE

Womack, Thomas, M, 30s, Euro-American, holistic medicine M.D.

Woodruff, Mitchell, M, 30s, Euro-American, biomedical researcher

Wright, Charlotte, F, 20s, Euro-American, Franklin, fast-food restaurant worker

Young, Saundra, F, 40s, African-American, day-care operator

APPENDIX 3

Questions for Neighborhood Interviews

_____

Background

How long have you lived in this neighborhood?
Who lives in the same household with you?
What occupations do people in your household have?

Neighborhood/Community

Would you tell me something about this neighborhood, what you like
    or don't like about it, what kinds of people live here? How is it sim-
    ilar to or different from other Baltimore neighborhoods?
Are you concerned about any controversial issues or debates that have
    directly affected your neighborhood recently (housing, zoning,
    schooling, traffic, crime, etc.)?

General Health

Do you do anything special in the way of diet or exercise for the sake
    of your health?
Is what you do now different from what you did some years ago or what
    your parents encouraged you to do when you were growing up?
What have you heard or seen about the immune system lately?
    Magazines, TV, etc.
What is your own understanding of how this system works and what it
    includes?

Do you do anything special (diet, exercise, etc.) for the benefit of your immune system?

Do you think your mother and father, or grandmother and grandfather, thought about the immune system?

Do you remember the polio epidemic of the 1940s and 1950s? What do you remember about it? What precautions did people take against polio before there was a vaccine? Do you remember hearing why they did these things? What is your understanding of how vaccines work?

Do you take any precautions when you are sick [or for your children if they are sick] to prevent others from getting the same illness?

Have you heard about the recommendation that everyone up to teenagers should get another measles vaccination? Do you plan to take any action on this? Why do you think it would be necessary?

What is your opinion on the amount of time and energy that scientists are devoting to understanding the human gene and to finding the genetic causes of diseases? Do you think there is any connection between understanding the human gene and understanding the immune system?

What do you imagine is happening inside your body when you start to catch a cold? in someone with arthritis? in someone with AIDS? What would you say happens in your body when you are exposed to some contagious illness and do not get it?

Do you think that one's state of mind or emotions can affect one's health? the immune system?

Have you heard of autoimmune diseases? How would you explain what they are?

What do you make of these photographs of:

- white blood cells and an asbestos fiber?
- white blood cells and bacteria?
- T cells and cancer cells?
- T cells and bacteria?

Does it change the way you think about yourself or your body to hear there are these things going on inside you?

HIV/AIDS

Have you heard any accounts about the origins of the virus that causes AIDS? Do any of these make sense to you?

What do you think the course of the disease is going to be in our country? in the world?

What do you think about the issue of testing people's blood for antibodies to HIV, the virus that can cause AIDS? Did your opinion about this change after the finding that a drug (AZT) can prolong the time before a person with HIV comes down with symptoms of AIDS?

How contagious do you think AIDS is? How do you think a person is most likely to come down with it? Do any other ways seem possible to you?

Do you think there is any difference in how likely men or women would be to catch it?

What would be your understanding of how AIDS babies get AIDS?

Do you think very much about this new "risk" in our lives?

Do you think children with AIDS should attend school as usual?

Do you think a cure for AIDS will be found? What form would it be likely to take?

How would you respond to this kind of statement from earlier in the epidemic: "The poor homosexuals, they have declared war on nature and now nature is exacting an awful retribution" (Patrick Buchannan).

How would you explain to a child how the immune system works or what AIDS is? Would you draw a picture of your conception of the immune system?

What would you say is the difference between AIDS and cancer?

General

What is your feeling about how well the Baltimore area is doing in social or economic terms now as compared to, say, ten or twenty years ago?

What is your feeling about how well the United States is doing in social or economic terms today as compared to the past?

End

What did you think of the interview?

Would you mind if we contacted you again in a year or so for a much briefer follow-up on any changes in your thinking that might occur?

NOTES

Part One: INTRODUCTION

1. Latour (1986) is perhaps his strongest statement about the power of science to affect the world. For a description of the interactions among scientists, fishermen, and scallops, see Callon (1986). Star (1991) points out the managerial or entrepreneurial assumptions in the actor network theory of Latour and Callon and suggests alternatives.

2. On the controversy as it erupted at the annual meeting of the American Anthropological Association, see Conkin (1992) and Coughlin (1992).

3. Recently in medical anthropology, attention has been drawn to the importance of taking into account the experiences of those who are suffering with illness as a way of understanding the "lived, felt quality of human events" (Ware 1992:357).

4. For an exploration of the problems inherent in taking the exposition of the experiences of a repressed group as the goal of analysis, see Scott (1992:25): "Making visible the experience of a different group exposes the existence of repressive mechanisms, but not their inner workings or logics."

5. For other sources on the new genetics, see Duster (1990), Holtzman (1989), and Lewontin (1991).

6. It is the history of the term *configuration* in anthropology (Linton's [1936] configuration of culture) and computer science (configuration of the system) that I want to draw on here.

7. "The United States' distribution of income in the 1980s can be likened to Hirschman's . . . famous tunnel at rush hour. One lane, representing the incomes of highly paid workers and capitalists, is moving ahead rapidly. Another lane, representing the incomes of the majority of families, is barely creeping along" (Gramich, Kasten, and Sammartino 1993:225).

267

8. For a selection of people the Clinton campaign brought into the foreground, see Reich (1991), Osborne and Gaebler (1992), or Marshall and Schram (1993).

Part Two: HISTORICAL OVERVIEW

1. On the way nostalgia works in and against social theory, see Robertson (1992) and Strathern (in press).

2. NORC provided us with the original questionnaires from this survey for Maryland, immediately contiguous states to the north and south, as well as southern New England. The study was called "Attitudes, Information and Customary Behavior in Health Matters" (NORC Study 367, 1955). It was based on a national probability sample.

3. On the anxieties about domestic sanitation in the late nineteenth century, see Tomes (1990).

4. Sanitarians in the late nineteenth century were concerned that the germ theory of disease might restrict the moral field of public health action (Rosenberg 1979a; Stevenson 1955).

5. For a comparative treatment of the importance of bacteriology to public health at this time in the United States and England, see Fee and Porter (1992).

6. On how in polio epidemics in the early decades of the twentieth century links were made between polio, dirt, and the immigrant poor, see Rogers (1992).

7. Ritchie continued to publish and reprint his books on sanitation and physiology into the 1940s (e.g., Ritchie 1948).

8. Seltzer (1992) is a rewarding exploration of the implications of the widespread use of machine-body imagery in art and literature in the early twentieth century.

9. College textbooks of a slightly earlier era frequently describe the body as being made up of "systems": the skeletal system, the muscular system, the nervous system, or the reproductive system (Kimber, Gray, and Stackpole 1934:11). For ideas in nineteenth-century America about health and disease as holistic, interactive, and integrating mind and body in a balanced whole, see Rosenberg 1979b, 1983, 1989). Tomes (1990:522–23) discusses how the hygiene of the late nineteenth century focused on providing pure "intake" (clean water, food, and air) and effective removal of the "outgo" (respired air and waste matter). For a literary reference, see H. G. Wells's The War of the Worlds, in which the Martians were finally "slain by the putrefactive and disease bacteria against which their systems were unprepared" (Wells 1986:191).

It is important to note the differences between these notions about the "system" and contemporary notions of the body as a complex system. The earlier model tended to be a homeostatic one, in which the body changed from balance (health) to imbalance (sickness). In the contemporary model, as we will see, the body *in health* moves from one temporary disequilibrium to another, like an acrobat on a high wire. Canguilhem (1988:81–102) develops the genealogy of the concept of biological regulation in the eighteenth and nineteenth centuries.

10. I have discussed this further in Martin (1992). See also Gramsci (1971) and Wren (1979:7).

11. The literature on American society in the years after the Second World War is immense. For an overview, see Tuchman (1991). May (1988) focuses on the cultural meanings given at the time to women and sexuality; Jackson (1985) details the development of American suburbs.

12. I am struck by the emphasis in these first aid measures on the outer surfaces of the body, even though the danger is radioactive materials. First aid emphasizes putting on clean clothes, bathing, and scrubbing hard with soap, especially the hair and fingernails. The effects of radiation are acknowledged, but minimized: "you need not worry about lingering radioactivity after an air burst"; the effects of a ground or water burst are not always fatal (Pomeranz and Koll 1957:527–29).

13. Sometimes the body is aided in this by new "miracle drugs," especially antibiotics, that allow astonishingly rapid recovery from previously devastating diseases. For a general history of the development of antibiotics, see Wainwright (1990). For essays on the scientists who discovered them, see Moberg and Cohn (1990).

14. Unless otherwise noted, quotes from interviews are from transcriptions of tape recordings. Ellipses indicate brief omitted material; reduplicated words and phrases have been deleted without ellipses. Interviewers' questions and comments are italicized; explanatory interpolations are placed within brackets.

15. The term *flexible specialization* was first used in Piore and Sabel (1984).

16. For a different analysis of the relation between the global division of labor and flexible specialization, see Piore and Sabel (1984).

17. Noyelle and Stanback (1984:53ff.) classify Baltimore among cities in the United States as a "regional nodal diversified service center."

18. During 1992, Maryland had the fifth worst job loss in the nation, and Baltimore City bore the brunt of it (Clark 1993). Newspapers in late 1992 reported that "prospects for Maryland economy are grim" (Sarris 1992:1).

19. Rouse (1984) is an enthusiastic description of what urban redevelopment has meant for Baltimore by the chairman of the Rouse Co. which developed the festival marketplace at the Inner Harbor in 1980.

20. On how the Inner Harbor development has brought low-paying service jobs and a net flow of profits and public funds out of the city, see Harvey (1991b:240).

21. Zukin (1991b:29–38) contains an enlightening discussion of *Red Baker* and other novels that depict postmodern urban landscapes.

Chapter 1: The Body at War

1. According to *Magazine Index*, there were about thirty articles on some aspect of immunity or the immune system published per year from 1960 to 1980.

2. Peter Jaret, interview, December 1992. The details were kindly provided by the National Geographic Society.

3. This magazine is translated into sixteen languages.

4. According to a count produced by *Magazine Index*, by 1981–85 there were over 150 articles a year, by 1986–90 over 300 per year, and in 1992 alone over 450.

5. Films for the Humanities and Sciences, *1992–93 Health Education Video Catalogue* (Princeton, N.J.).

6. For descriptions, see Copeland (1992) and Rubin (1989).

7. Mind Matters Seminars (Stanford, Calif.) ran three seminars on "The Immune System: Minding the Body, Embodying the Mind" in the Baltimore area in the fall of 1992.

8. The Johns Hopkins School of Continuing Studies ran a course on psychoneuroimmunology in the fall of 1991 that was oversubscribed; the course was offered again the following year.

9. Haraway (1989:14) terms this the "hierarchical, localized organic body." In her work, Haraway eloquently stresses the displacement of the hierarchical, localized body by new parameters: "a highly mobile field of strategic differences . . . a semiotic system, a complex meaning-producing field" (p. 15). No one could improve on her characterization of these new elements; I would add only that there may be strategic reasons why a remnant of the old body is carried forward with the new.

10. This may relate to what Petchesky (1981:208) calls the ideology of "privatism."

11. For lack of space, I cannot deal with the subtleties of how this "old body discourse" appears in interviews. Suffice it to say that military metaphors are extremely widespread.

12. These include mass media magazines such as *Time* and *Newsweek* as well as the *National Geographic*. They also include more expensive items such as Lennert Nilsson's popular coffee table book *The Body Victorious* (1985).

13. At times the "police" become more like antiterrorist squads, as befits the task of finding enemies within who are bent on destruction. Paula Treichler points out that the AIDS virus is a "spy's spy, capable of any deception . . . a terrorist's terrorist, an Abu Nidal of viruses" (1987:282).

14. Overheard by Paula Treichler, personal communication.

15. B cells are not always feminized: Michaud and Feinstein (1989:13, 7, respectively) depict them as admirals and supermen.

16. For a lengthy discussion of why teamwork and group cooperation are required in the economic world, see Kash (1989).

17. Keller (1992:116–17) illustrates how easily the language of evolutionary biology slips from descriptions of nature as neutrally indifferent to descriptions of nature as callous and hostile.

18. Elsewhere, I am developing an account of fetus-mother interaction in an immunological environment in which blurry self-nonself discrimination is assumed. After all, babies are born, tissue can be grafted, and many bacteria live (to the benefit of our health) in our gut.

19. This pamphlet can be obtained by calling 1-800-4CANCER or through Info-quest (CD-ROM) in many public libraries.

20. A Toronto newspaper reported that "Vancouver psychologist Andrew Feldmar offers an intriguing explanation for the adult onset of autoimmune disease: 'It strikes people who in their childhood were inhibited from differentiating who is their enemy, who is their friend'" (Maté 1993:16).

21. Reported to me by Ariane van der Straten.

22. David Napier explores the implications of using a metaphor of self-destruction to describe illness. He suggests that, despite the disorientation that might be produced, telling someone who is suffering that her body is at war with itself can be a helpful thing to do: "People often do feel better when they can salvage a 'self' from a ravaged body; we learn to deal with illness by setting it up as something against which we can define (even through dissociation) a better condition of selfhood" (1992:187).

23. For a detailed discussion of Baudrillard's views of the media, see Connor (1989). I have found Mah (1991) useful in considering the pitfalls of thinking that any text can be treated as a transparent window into culture. Recent ethnographic media studies have allowed the "reading" of media messages to take into account what people in the culture say (e.g., Morley 1992). For some of the rich variety of current studies of culture through the media, see Gitlin (1987), Fiske (1987), and Robbins (1993).

Chapter 2: Immunology on the Street

1. When the graduate students and I conducted interviews, we often displayed lively enthusiasm for the interesting things that people said. However, we all tried to avoid encouraging certain kinds of expressions and discouraging others. Presumably, in this interview, if Arthur Harrison had described the body as a mechanical device, the interviewer would have showed just as much interest.

Chapter 3: "Fix My Head"

1. Important studies by anthropologists of the culture of alternative medicine in the United States include Crawford (1980) and McGuire (1988).

2. From a study of literature from the new age community, Andrew Ross concludes that "non-legitimate scientific cultures, no matter how esoteric, unavoidably bear the impress of the dominant orthodoxy's language" (1991:30). Alternative scientific cultures share with mainstream science an emphasis on the interconnectedness of systems.

3. It would lead me too far afield to elaborate it here, but immune system discourse also allows practitioners to build a bridge between the "old cities" of alternative medicine (the body as composed of humors or ch'i and the "new suburbs" (the body as composed of scientifically linked neurological, cognitive, vascular, etc. systems). Thanks to Lorna Rhodes for pointing this out to me.

4. A comprehensive sourcebook of recent work in psychoneuroimmunology is Ader, Felten, and Cohen (1991).

5. In the spring of 1993, after the period of our research, the five-part television series "Healing and the Mind," narrated by Bill Moyers, aired on PBS, focusing on the immune system, psychoneuroimmunology, Chinese medicine, and many other alternative therapies. (The series also appeared in book form [see Moyers 1993].) This program followed by only a few months the establishment at the National Institutes of Health of the new Office of Alternative Medicine (Angier 1993).

Chapter 4: Immunophilosophy

1. Gane (1991:130ff.) discusses the more complex senses in which Baudrillard uses the term *implosion*.

2. About two years later, I was to see a biologist make this same hand gesture on the television special "Healing and the Mind." Candace Pert was explaining how peptides work: "Peptides, receptors, cells. The receptors are dynamic. They're wiggling, vibrating energy molecules that are not only changing their shape from millisecond to millisecond, but actually changing what they're coupled to. One moment they're coupled up to one protein in the membrane, and the next moment they can couple up to another. It's a very dynamic, fluid system" (Pert 1993:186). Enthusiastic descriptions of the enormous flexibility of the immune system are also frequently found in the scientific literature (see, e.g., Cohen 1987:54).

3. Valentine (1967) contains photographs of the very micrographs that Edelman saw.

4. On the isolated, compulsive, competitive world of men that characterizes work in high-energy physics and computer science, see Traweek (1988) and Wajcman (1991:141–49).

5. On the important role that mobilizing a wide variety of research materials played in the development of early twentieth-century reproductive biology, see Clarke (1987). Charlesworth et al. (1989: 148ff.) has an enlightening discussion of an Australian immunology department's involvement with raw materials as well as machinery in generating data.

6. His wordplay was in the mode of the many compound terms in the scientific literature beginning with *immuno-*, from *immunoarchitecture* to *immunovisualization*.

7. Karush (1989:78–79) has an illuminating discussion of military metaphors in immunology. Mazumdar (1975) traces the early history of immunity as the body's armed struggle against a foreign enemy back to the influence of the Darwinian survival of the fittest in the 1890s.

8. Published references to antibodies as "tailor-made" are not uncommon (see, e.g., Folkers 1993:1).

9. Rouse (1993) reviews some important implications of the heterogeneity of the sciences.

Chapter 5: Complex Systems

1. Katherine Hayles has explored what she calls the "archipelago of chaos" as it emerges in science, contemporary fiction, and poststructuralism. Her task is to describe the "broader cultural conditions that authorize the new visions of chaos," to trace how influence "spreads out through a diffuse network of everyday experiences," creating "a cultural field within which certain questions or concepts become highly charged" (1990:3, 4).

2. For other anthropological engagements with chaos theory, see Abrahams (1990), Brown (1992), and Cheater (1993).

3. Within biology and medicine generally, many other fields are also experimenting with applications of chaos theory — e.g., cardiology (Skinner 1993), neurology (Molnar and Skinner 1992), genetics (Oliver et al. 1993), nursing (Coppa 1993), and psychiatry (Schmid 1991), to mention only a few.

4 The huge international success of *Jurassic Park* — the movie, the original book by Michael Crichton (1990), and other spin-off books — happened just after the period of my research. It is interesting to speculate how the plot line's reliance on chaos theory might have increased or deepened many people's awareness of the nature of complex systems. Gould (1993) discusses the accuracy of the chaos theory used in Crichton's book and the caricature of chaos theory that appears in the movie.

5. In *Wonderful Life* (1989), Stephen Jay Gould stresses the role of tiny accidents early in history that affected the outcome of evolution more than the relative "fitness" of different life forms.

6. Laura Nader (1990:291ff.) provides a comparative and historical discussion of the variety of ways in which an ideology of harmony has been used and resisted.

Chapter 6: System Breakdown

1. Because this chapter takes a particular approach to HIV/AIDS, I do not refer to the bulk of the extensive literature on its cultural and social significance. On AIDS activists and research science, see Treichler (1991). On the cultural construction of AIDS, see Patton (1990). On the historical construction of AIDS, see Fee and Fox (1992).

2. Doubt about the adequacy of the current paradigm was expressed at the conference itself. In his opening remarks, Jonathan Mann referred to "our current vision of AIDS" as "outdated" and a "straightjacket" (Mann 1992:6–7). Laury Oaks attended the conference for our group.

3. Duesberg explains his theory in, e.g., Duesberg (1988, 1991). On Sonnabend's earlier contributions, see Sonnabend, Witkin, and Purtilo (1984).

4. As recently as 1989, it was said that a conference on AIDS vaccine development marked the giving way of pessimism to cautious optimism, that "the fundamental focus had changed from 'if a vaccine could be developed' to 'when'" (Glass et al. 1990:413).

5. The views that question the current paradigm in AIDS research have been appearing in less visible locations for some time. See Palca (1991), Duesberg (1991), and the extensive references in pts. 1 and 2 of Root-Bernstein (1992). For a discussion of the early disputes over the identification and naming of HIV, see Treichler (1992).

6. A subject that needs more attention than I can give it here is the connection between the notion that the body is at war in its fight against microbes and the notion that microbiologists are warriors who can come to the aid of the body. In one newspaper account, AIDS virologists are depicted as "a breed apart, eager to roll up their sleeves, get down in there, into the middle of the warfare, engage in hand-to-hand combat with the enemy. . . . Like everyone who has ever fought in a war, you have to be able to handle the moments of terror and failure" (Carton 1993:53). This heroic role for scientists is buttressed by the idea that there is one clearly identifiable cause of AIDS, HIV. Even though HIV is "wily" and "evil," it can potentially be vanquished if scientists are clever and persistent enough.

7. Very important work is being done on the way the "body at war" model can be deployed as a part of homophobia by Catherine Waldby of Macquarie

University. In her account, the homosexual body invites its own destruction by being too permeable, both to viruses and to other bodies.

8. The mass media tends to position its audience as largely immune witnesses to the disaster of AIDS, people who can safely watch it from outside. Art produced about AIDS tends to position its audience as people who are directly implicated in the epidemic, who are in danger, or already infected, inside it (Goldstein 1991:20–21).

Chapter 7: Flexible Systems

1. I argue that flexibility is a trait that has recently become intensely desirable in a general way, but not that it has never been cultivated by anyone before. Rhoda Halperin (1990) shows how the rural poor in Kentucky have for some time been flexibly making use of multiple kinds of work, economies, and production, within the purview of the family network, to provide themselves a livelihood. Although the rural and urban poor may have been using such flexible strategies for many generations, there is something different about the flexibility that is now broadly enjoined. As Sheldon Wolin puts it, "Conceptions of change are also susceptible to change." What he says of "change" is as true of "flexibility": "For an 'advanced society' struggling amidst the rigors of the international economy, change is necessary for survival. It must, therefore, be produced as a matter of deliberate policy" (1989: 77).

2. Whether employees actually comply or resist depends on many factors, including whether they are unionized.

3. Many analysts are very critical of the concept of flexible specialization, arguing that it is a "fetish" that dazzles our eyes and conceals from us the real processes of oppression that are going on (Pollert 1991; see also Smith 1991; and Nolan and O'Donnell 1991). The collection edited by Stephen Wood (1989) is a careful, critical examination of the implications of flexible specialization. Garrahan and Stewart (1993) is a workers'-eye view of working in a Nissan manufacturing plant, which places an extraordinary stress on the virtues of flexibility, teamwork, and quality.

4. Freeman (1993) discusses some of the social and economic effects of deunionization during the 1980s.

5. All are contained in the newspapers listed in the *National Newspaper Index*.

6. The term *flexible weapons* appears in the subject coding system of the *National Newspaper Index*. See, e.g., Wren (1991).

7. This is only one of many areas in which scientists investigating the molecular properties of proteins and nucleic acids are realizing that these molecules are mechanically flexible. A recent article on the "moltenness" or "squidgeability" of intrinsic membrane proteins closes by linking the flexibil-

ity of these proteins to the flexibility of the NatWest credit card (see fig. 23 above): "There may be something of fundamental significance in the fact that a well-known credit card was advertised as 'your flexible friend'" (Pain 1991:354).

8. The flexible, fluid, accommodating self is found much earlier in psychology, e.g., in Carl Rogers's *Client-Centered Therapy* (1951).

9. Or see Chapman (1992:49): "The transition to a new era beyond the Cold War will require an adroit, flexible, and forward-looking leader."

Part Five: PRACTICUMS

1. Barbara Stafford argues that the eighteenth-century mode of keeping in touch with the world — "the full and well-rounded experiencing of things . . . interlocking the observer with the plastic, limitless, and heterogeneous flux of the environment" — can provide the basis for a mode of perception suited to the present, in which "the public has to be educated to tackle multisensory problems. Inventiveness and flexibility in the automated workplace depend on a familiarity with many interconnected and different types of operations" (1991:476).

Chapter 8: Interpreting Electron Micrographs

1. For a description of high-energy physicists' use of slides in lectures, see Traweek (1992:429). For a description of how scientists use electron microscopy to convince their colleagues, see Rasmussen (1992).

2. For different views of the primacy of visual evidence in science, see Latour (1986) and Keller and Grontkowski (1983).

3. On how electron micrographs are made into "docile objects" in the laboratory, see Lynch (1985). We will see below that nonscientists find micrographs distancing. To the extent that the painstaking labor of producing the specimens and taking the photographs is done by technicians instead of research scientists, the scientists are also, in this sense, distanced from micrographs.

4. For a few of the many instances, see micrographs that appear in the *Economist* ("A Day for AIDS?" 1988), *Nutrition Action* (Barone 1988), *Healthsharing* (Elliott 1989), and the *New Yorker* (Preston 1992).

5. For the most part, electron micrographs occur in the domain of the "media" rather than in clinical contexts. Hence, although they often depict biological processes that are central to human health and illness, if they are interpreted at all, it is not usually in the presence of or with the help of a medical practitioner.

6. Interview with Richard Preston, 28 April 1993.

7. Studies of the popular media that solicit reactions from viewers have been criticized for inciting responses that might not occur if the subjects were simply watching television in their living room (Modleski 1991:38). Our procedure is subject to the same criticism. However, we were soliciting a response not to just any mass media but to media representations of scientific knowledge. Given how hegemonic such knowledge is often taken to be, it seemed a legitimate question whether people would be willing to interpret it under any circumstances.

8. In an example taken from contemporary science, Cambrosio and Keating (1992:370, 365) detail how new entities, monoclonal antibodies, and an associated machine, a fluorescence-activated cell sorter (FACS), came into standard usage in contemporary immunology. These tools were involved in a circular process of constituting standard techniques at the same time as they were sources of standardization.

9. Bjorn Claeson undertook this project.

Chapter 9: Saturation

1. Six years of drought in California have provided conditions favorable to the growth and spread of the fungus that causes valley disease. People with poorer immune responses are more vulnerable.

2. One woman wrote a letter to the editor about an article on whether doctors should reveal terminal diagnoses to their patients. She did not wish such information from her doctor, she said, because, "the more I knew, the more anxious I would become, thereby causing further stress to my immune system" (*New York Times Magazine*, 14 February 1993, 8).

3. On cancer, see Fisher (1991) and Kolata (1992). On transplants, see Rosenthal (1989) and "Immunex Advances in Bid" (1990).

4. For a review of the development of scientific knowledge about connections between the nervous system and the immune system, see Janković (1989).

5. The Disney Corp. would not quote any figures on attendance at "Body Wars" because, they told me, they regard this as proprietary information. Guidebooks, as well as general lore, stress both the long wait for this ride because of its popularity and its turbulence: cars often have to be hosed out after use because people have vomited in them. Monica Schoch-Spana went on this ride on behalf of our research.

6. Other computer games about the immune system are "The Immune System: Your Magic Doctor" (Rubin 1989) and "The Immune System: Our Internal Defender" (Copeland 1992).

7. Omega Institute's 1993 catalog lists a workshop by Paul Pearsall called "Intimacy and Immunity."

8. "The labour which is uniformly materialised in them must be uniform, homogeneous, simple labour; it matters as little whether this is embodied in gold, iron, wheat or silk, as it matters to oxygen whether it is found in rusty iron, in the atmosphere, in the juice of grapes or in human blood. But digging gold, mining iron, cultivating wheat and weaving silk are qualitatively different kinds of labour. In fact, what appears objectively as diversity of the use-values, appears, when looked at dynamically, as diversity of the activities which produce those use-values. . . . Different use-values are, moreover, products of the activity of different individuals and therefore the result of individually different kinds of labour. But as exchange-values they represent the same homogeneous labour, i.e., labour in which the individual characteristics of the workers are obliterated. Labour which creates exchange-value is thus *abstract general* labour" (Marx [1859] 1970:29).

9. A single-topic issue of the *Scientific American* is scheduled to appear in September 1993 (vol. 29, no. 3), just as this book goes to press. Its title, "Life, Death, and the Immune System," evokes the sort of extension of the immune system to embrace everything that I am describing.

10. Paul Ansa raised this question at York University.

11. Thomas Moench, M.D., was especially helpful.

Chapter 10: Educating and Training the Body

1. For a scientific account of the thymus as an educational institution, see Sell (1987:57).

2. For a model of cancer therapy that is called "teaching the immune system to fight cancer," see Boon (1993).

3. Criticism of vaccines was not uncommon in the earlier part of the century, but it focused mostly on problems caused by undue haste in production or the complications of corporate involvement in scientific research (Rogers 1992:180–85). Today, physicians are reported to be "rebelling" against public health and medical society recommendations to vaccinate children against hepatitis B (Rosenthal 1993b). A major controversy has erupted among medical scientists over the value of the forthcoming vaccine for chicken pox (Rosenthal 1993a). On the popular front, *Mothering* magazine published a book, *Vaccinations: the Rest of the Story* (O'Mara 1992), reprinting articles and letters written between 1979 and 1992, most of which are highly skeptical of the value of childhood immunizations.

4. John Guillory provides an important analysis of the American school as an institution that "regulates and thus distributes cultural capital *unequally*. The largest context for analyzing the school as an institution is therefore the

reproduction of the social order, with all of its various inequities" (1993:ix). The connections between wealth and education, which Guillory points out are seldom analyzed, are made at least rhetorically clear in the recent emphasis on continuing education and retraining for employees: it is now your responsibility as an employee to invest in your own education, build up a "portfolio of up-to-date skills" and "an endowment of flexible skills" (Richman 1993:58, 60).

5. Sometimes HIV is described as adapting to the human body much like an animal species occupying a new continent. This has been called being in "evolutionary fast-forward" (Bylinsky 1992:104).

6. In general, the scientists we interviewed assumed that state-sponsored vaccination programs were a good thing. One need only look at discussions of research to develop better vaccines, however, to see how many are the health consequences of using vaccines and how complex the calculation of acceptable risk (Ellis 1992). Vaccines for whooping cough (pertussis), e.g., have a great many shortcomings from the point of view of scientists trying to develop a better vaccine (Brennan et al. 1992).

7. This finding is discussed fully in Martin et al. (in press). The extent to which this group — almost all African-American men — is actually involved with the prison system was made clear by a study published while we were conducting our research: "In Baltimore, more than half of the 60,715 black males, ages 18 to 35, were under the supervision of the criminal justice system on an average day in 1991" (West 1992:1).

Chapter 11: Educating and Training at Work

1. This chapter deals with only a small portion of the research that I have conducted on work and community restructuring and on new conceptions of management. I am planning a second volume that will expand what I say here and in addition explore changes in the concept and practice of bureaucratic organization as well as gender definitions in the workplace. The use of "soft" disciplines like cultural anthropology to bring about change in the "culture" of the workplace is central to what is going on.

2. Because I am planning an extended discussion of work reorganization in another context, I do not provide complete references to the relevant literature. One particularly interesting sociological analysis is Sewell and Wilkinson (1992).

3. The literature on restructuring the corporation is immense. An early classic is Drucker (1989). Books on or by three of the early figures in the field are Crosby (1984), Juran (1988), and Walton (1986). Recent monographs are Drucker (1992) and Hiam (1992). A book explaining the Clinton administration's endorsement of many of these ideas is Marshall and Schram (1993).

4. For some of the variety, see Juran (1988), Crosby (1984), and Deming (1993).

5. TQM has recently been sanctioned and promulgated by the Conference Board, a network of major companies and executives in fifty countries (Hiam 1992).

6. Among many related activities at my university was "Workforce 2000 v. Hopkins Workplace 2000," a conference held in September 1992. On quality programs for educational institutions, see "Visions of Excellence" (1993). On applying quality initiatives to government, see Osborne and Gaebler (1992).

7. This came on the heels of a recession that caused alarm among the ranks of those promoting TQM. At the end of 1992, there were reports in the mainstream press that business had "soured" on TQM, citing a survey by Rath and Strong that showed how most American firms were found lacking on quality criteria (Mathews 1992). But, in the TQM journals, this was given a very different interpretation. There the survey was quoted as concluding that "there will be no long-term future without a formal quality effort. . . . Our survey shows there's still a huge gap in understanding how to achieve 'total quality'" ("Total Quality Report Card" 1992). By early 1993 there were reports in the press that, following one of the central procedures of TQM, President Clinton "hired management experts . . . to hold team-building sessions . . . at Camp David for his Cabinet and other high-ranking officials" (Baer 1993:1).

8. This principle is often stated in the TQM literature, but, in practice, work and life managed under TQM often seem similar in central respects to scientific management in the era of Taylor and Ford. Roberts and Sergesketter (1993:50), applying TQM to personal tasks and goals, happily claim that they can reduce the time it takes to shave by three minutes! Thus was scientific management applied to home life in *Cheaper by the Dozen* (Gilbreth and Carey 1948).

9. With the huge popularity of his methods in the United States in the 1980s and 1990s, Deming worries that a flow of ideas and practices back to Japan might "infect" Japanese industry with American "diseases": "It is important that Japanese management remain strong, not weakened and diluted by adoption of some of the practices that are largely responsible for the decline of western industry. It is possible for a strong body to become infected, to become weak. Japanese management has responsibilities to continue to be strong and not to pick up infections from western management" (Walton 1986:248).

10. Corporate America spent $45.5 billion in 1990 on training and development. About half of 1 percent of that total, or $227 million, is now spent on experience-based training, and this figure is expected to increase significantly in the next five years (Laabs 1991:56). On the basis of a survey conducted by the Association for Training and Development, it was reported that, despite the devastation experienced by the ranks of middle managment during the

period of our research, "corporate trainers are escaping the layoff ax." And "nearly three-fourths of the training executives expected their budgets to rise next year" ("Corporate Trainers Manage to Keep Jobs" 1992:1).

11. In an ad for Chemical Bank, a woman sailor makes it clear to men rowers, "Be innovative or be gone," demonstrating the kind of gender reversal being called for in today's business environment (*Business Week*, 28 December/4 January 1993, 76–77). An amazingly precise reversal of this image was used in a poster, "Handicapped!" for women's suffrage in nineteenth-century England (Tickner 1988). In this poster, the positions of men and women are the reverse of the Chemical Bank version: a woman rows laboriously in an unsuccessful effort to keep up with a man sailing far ahead in a sailboat.

12. This aspect of training on ropes courses has been used directly to sell commodities. An ad for Saturn in the *Economist* (10 November 1990) read: "One thing we do, as a team-building exercise, is each of us straps on mountaineering gear, climbs up a pole and jumps off. *People ask, "What does jumping off a forty-foot pole have to do with building a car?"* Well, I'm the kind of guy who doesn't even want to stand on a chair. But there I was, forty feet up, and four people holding a rope are keeping me from breaking my neck. Two assembly line technicians, an engineer and a finance guy. That's when it really hits you what Saturn means when they talk about partnership. 'Cause you know it won't be a very pleasant landing if only a couple of people are doing their job. Funny, the things you have to go through to build a better car. . . . "

13. Mark Sandler is not the only trainer who relies on the immune system as a teaching device. Philip Crosby, a prolific writer and consultant on quality, and formerly in charge of quality within ITT, recommends that companies should administer a "quality vaccine." This training program will be sure to produce "antibodies" to the most common impediments in the way of achieving quality management (Crosby 1984:6–7). Crosby's prescription is quoted in a recent book intended to carry TQM into the business community in Great Britain (Munro-Faure and Munro-Faure 1992:290).

14. Wendy Richardson attended the workshop for our group.

15. It is an intriguing question why two conservative philanthropists would be interested in experiential education.

16. In another context, I plan to write about the complex mix of power, resource sharing, and risk sharing that these plans seem to entail.

Part Six: POST-DARWINISM

1. Some of the major sources on social Darwinism in the nineteenth century are Bannister (1979) and Hofstadter ([1959] 1992). A particularly important collection of articles on how these ideas worked in colonial practice is Breman (1990).

2. Disease is only one of the apocalyptic disasters that threaten us as we approach the millennium. On how the world might end with a collision of an asteroid or a comet, see Begley (1992).

3. It is interesting that Richard Preston, the author of the article on Ebola virus, is also the author of a book on astrophysics that devotes considerable attention to astrophysical apocalypse, in the form of possible collisions of "near-earth objects" with the earth (see Preston 1987).

4. Another area that I am exploring elsewhere is the current alarm over the rise of infections that are resistant to antibiotics, e.g., certain strains of tuberculosis. See the series of articles that began with Specter (1992).

5. Marcellino's fears are not exaggerated, according to a study conducted under the auspices of the National Research Council. The study's conclusion was that HIV/AIDS is settling into "spatially and socially isolated groups and possibly becoming endemic within them" (Jonsen and Stryker 1993:7). The publication of this study was greeted by local Baltimore AIDS activists with scorn: "What it does is basically say the populations that are affected are of no consequence, are throwaways, and why bother with them. In a society where we claim to value everybody's life, that's exactly the opposite of what we ought to be telling people" (Gerstenzang 1993:13). Lorna Rhodes has pointed out to me that the "unhealthy," whether poor or rich, who have not become fit are an unending source of employment for people in many areas, from international development, health policy, and education, to therapy, corrections, and medicine. Their job consists in helping or forcing others to change themselves in order to attain a better, healthier self.

6. Similar evaluations are also found in technical scientific literature (see Solomon 1987). The work of Gerald Edelman has developed the idea that evolution, the brain, and the immune system all operate according to fundamentally similar Darwinian principles of natural selection (see Pagels 1989:136; Edelman 1987).

7. The complexities of New Age thought, and the ways it is distinguished from alternative medicine, are beyond the scope of my study. For useful introductions to the New Age, see Lewis and Melton (1992) and Hess (1993).

8. See Reich (1992:271–78) for a particularly cogent desciption of how new communities of like incomes are developing in the U.S. in the late twentieth century. The wealthier communities are producing separate enclaves that close their borders against other, poorer communities like Warren.

9. For different views of the way nineteenth-century biology related to theories of social evolution, see Bowler (1988) and Young (1985). For another account of how a version of social Darwinism is operating in the contemporary United States, see Duster (1990).

10. In other realms, Darwinian ideas of natural selection continue to be used to justify social differences (see Degler 1991; or Hubbard and Wald 1993). Hubbard and Wald focus on how genetics can be a basis for making evaluative distinctions among people, quoting as an example Daniel Koshland,

molecular biologist and editor-in-chief of *Science*: "Is there an argument against making superior individuals? Not superior morally, and not superior philosophically, just superior in certain skills: better at computers, better as musicians, better physically. As society gets more complex, perhaps it must select for individuals more capable of coping with its complex problems" (1993:156).

11. Stolcke (1993) explores insightfully the relation between contemporary sexist and racist ideology and different kinds of control exerted on women in different parts of the world: "Pro-natalist conceptive policies in the so-called First World and aggressive population control policies in the Third World are exemplary of this racist-cum-sexist ideology" (p. 37).

12. In addition to looking at biology working *in* culture, one important challenge facing us is to understand how culture itself, sometimes in the form of or with the aid of concepts straight out of anthropology, becomes an operator that produces difference. This would alert us to the role of *anthropology's* concepts in establishing hierarchies of living or dying bodies, women's bodies, or populations. This theme is central to the research that I am carrying out in corporations.

13. One early use of the hundredth monkey theory is in Keyes (1982). A skeptical review is in Amundson (1991).

14. Drawing out the implications of this purported disengagement from space would take me too far afield here. Elsewhere, I am considering these claims about space in relation to the kind of power that Foucault identified for an earlier era, a power that was contained by space and used it as a means of exerting discipline. On current theorizing about space, see Watts (1992).

15. According to Jameson (1984), postmodern forms reveal the "cultural logic" (p. 57) of late capitalism. They are a "figuration of . . . the whole world system of present-day multinational capitalism" (p. 79). They are an approach to a representation of a new reality, a peculiar new form of realism, a kind of mimesis of reality (p. 88). For Harvey (1989:344), these forms are also mimetic; "in the last instance," they are produced by the experience of time-space compression, itself the product of processes in flexible accumulation.

16. Michel Callon suggested this in conversations with me.

17. Obeyesekere (1990:56–57) discusses how the concept of overdetermination could be applied to symbolic forms.

18. A vast number of studies, following Foucault, see bodies as texts inscribed with marks of power. For some examples, see Scarry (1985), Rabinbach (1990), and Gusterson (1991).

19. In *The Feminist Case against Bureaucracy* (1984), e.g., Kathy Ferguson argues forcefully against the repression inherent in a hierarchical bureaucracy and embraces as a solution principles straight out of TQM. Arney (1991:147) discusses this.

20. On some of these effects, see Harvey (1991a:71) and Rustin (1989).

REFERENCES

Abrahams, R. 1990. Chaos and Kachin. *Anthropology Today* 6, no. 3:15–17.

Achterberg, J., and G. F. Lawlis. 1992. Imagery in healing workshop. Boulder, Colo.: Sounds True. Audiotape.

Ader, R., D. L. Felten, and N. Cohen, eds. 1991. *Psychoneuroimmunology*. 2d ed. San Diego, Calif.: Academic.

Ainsworth-Land, G. 1986. *Grow or die: The unifying principle of transformation*. New York: Wiley.

Alcohol intake and immunity. 1988. *Nutrition Today*, July, 33.

Alpers, S. 1983. *The art of describing: Dutch art in the seventeenth century*. Chicago: University of Chicago Press.

Altman, L. K. 1991. A White House puzzle: Immunity ailments: George and Barbara Bush have Graves' disease, their dog Millie has lupus — all autoimmune diseases. *New York Times*, 28 May, 1.

Amundson, R. 1991. The hundredth monkey phenomenon. In *The hundredth monkey and other paradigms of the paranormal*, ed. K. Frazier. Buffalo, N.Y.: Prometheus.

Anderson, R. M., and R. M. May. 1993. Understanding the AIDS pandemic. *Medicine: Special Issue of the Scientific American* 4, no. 1:86–92.

Anderson, W. T. 1993. Have we outgrown the age of heroes? *Utne Reader*, no. 57 (May): 95–100.

Angier, N. 1993. Where the unorthodox gets a hearing at N.I.H. *New York Times*, 16 March, 1.

Arens, W. 1979. *The man-eating myth: Anthropology and anthropophagy*. Oxford: Oxford University Press.

Arney, W. R. 1991. *Experts in the age of systems*. Albuquerque: University of New Mexico Press.

Attali, J. 1991. *Millennium: Winners and losers in the coming world order*. New York: Times Books.

Avrameas, S. 1991. Natural autoantibodies: From "horror autotoxicus" to "gnothi seauton." *Immunology Today* 12, no. 5 (May): 154–58.

Baer, S. 1993. A new age administration. *Baltimore Sun*, 7 February, 1.

Balibar, E. 1991a. Is there a "neo-racism"? In *Race, nation, class: Ambiguous identities,* ed. E. Balibar and I. Wallerstein. London: Verso.

———. 1991b. Preface. In *Race, nation, class: Ambiguous identities*, ed. E. Balibar and I. Wallerstein. London: Verso.

Bannister, R. C. 1979. *Social Darwinism: Science and myth in Anglo-American social thought*. Philadelphia: Temple University Press.

Banta, M. 1993. *Taylored lives: Narrative productions in the age of Taylor, Veblen, and Ford*. Chicago: University of Chicago Press.

Barone, J. 1988. Can diet protect your immune system? *Nutrition Action* 15, no. 6 (August): 3–7.

Bateson, G. 1972. *Steps to an ecology of mind*. New York: Ballantine.

Baudrillard, J. 1985. The masses: The implosion of the social in the media. *New Literary History* 16, no. 3 (March): 577–89.

Bauman, Z. 1992a. *Intimations of postmodernity*. London: Routledge.

———. 1992b. Survival as a cultural construct. In *Cultural theory and cultural change*, ed. M. Featherstone. London: Sage.

Begley, S. 1992. The science of doom. *Newsweek*, 23 November, 56–60.

Benedikt, M. 1991. Introduction. In *Cyberspace: First steps*, ed. M. Benedikt. Cambridge, Mass.: MIT Press

Benitez-Rojo, A. 1992. *The repeating island: The Caribbean and the postmodern perspective*. Durham, N.C.: Duke University Press.

Benziger, J. 1989. *The corpuscles: Adventures in innerspace*. Waterville, Maine: Corpuscles InterGalactica.

———. 1990. *The corpuscles meet the virus invaders*. Waterville, Maine: Corpuscles InterGalactica.

Berkow, I. 1992. Unspoken concerns about Magic. *New York Times*, 3 October, 31.

Bernsley, D. 1951. What to do during the polio season. *House Beautiful*, August, 6.

Bertalanffy, L. von. 1975. *Perspectives on general system theory: Scientific philosophical studies*. New York: Braziller.

Bhat, T. N., G. A. Bentley, T. O. Fischmann, and R. J. Poljak. 1990. Small rearrangements in structures of Fv and Fab fragments of antibody D1.3 on antigen binding. *Nature*, 347, no. 6292 (4 October): 483–85.

Bialkowski, C. 1991. Your best defense. *Weight Watcher's Magazine*, December, 16–18.

Bishop, J. E. 1988. Human immune system transplanted into mice successfully by Stanford team. *Wall Street Journal*, 15 September, 18.

———. 1990. Protein may limit damage in heart attacks, arthritis. *New York Times*, 13 July, 4.

Black, P. J. 1991. Turning off renegade T cells. *Business Week*, 18 November, 69.

Blakeslee, S. 1993. Mystery of sleep yields as studies reveal immune tie. *New York Times*, 3 August, 1, 6.

Bloch, M. 1991. Language, anthropology, and cognitive science. *Man* 26, no. 2:183–98.

Bodanis, D. 1986. *The secret house*. New York: Simon & Schuster.

Boon, T. 1993. Teaching the immune system to fight cancer. *Scientific American* 266, no. 3 (March): 82–89.

Borgmann, A. 1992. *Crossing the postmodern divide*. Chicago: University of Chicago Press.

Born, W., et al. 1990. Recognition of heat shock proteins and γ δ cell function. *Immunology Today* 11, no. 2 (February): 40–43.

Bourdieu, P. 1977. *Outline of a theory of practice*. Cambridge: Cambridge University Press.

Bower, B. 1987. Taking care of immunity. *Science News* 132, no. 11:168.

Bowler, P. J. 1988. *The non-Darwinian revolution: Reinterpreting a historical myth*. Baltimore: Johns Hopkins University Press.

Boyer, P. 1985. *By the bomb's early light: American thought and culture at the dawn of the atomic age*. New York: Pantheon.

Boyett, J. H., and H. P. Conn. 1991. *Workplace 2000: The revolution reshaping american business*. New York: Dutton.

Brallier, L. W. 1986. To your health. *Nation's Business* 74, no. 4:73.

Braly, J., E. R. Braverman, N. S. Orenstein, M. R. Werback, and C. B. Simone. 1992. How to achieve a healthy immune system: Advice from the experts. *Health News and Review* 2 (March): 18–19.

Brecher, R., and E. Brecher. 1954. Are we expecting too much too soon from the new polio vaccine? *Parents' Magazine*, July, 31–33, 72–74.

———. 1957. Why your body stays well. *Reader's Digest*, November, 122–26.

Breman, J., ed. 1990. *Imperial monkey business: Racial supremacy in social Darwinist theory and colonial practice*. Centre for Asian Studies Monographs, no. 3. Amsterdam: VU University Press.

Brennan, M. J., D. L. Burns, B. D. Meade, R. D. Shahin, and C. R. Manclark. 1992. Recent advances in the development of pertussis vaccines. In *Vaccines: New approaches to immunological problems*, ed. R. W. Ellis. Boston: Butterworth-Heinemann.

Brodeur, P. 1989. Annals of radiation: The hazards of electromagnetic fields, part 1. *New Yorker*, 12 June, 51–88.

Brody, J. E. 1989. Intriguing studies link nutrition to immunity. *New York Times*, 21 March, 1.

———. 1992. Researchers discover new therapies to avert repeated miscarriages; techniques based on fetal immunology are paying off. *New York Times,* 15 December, 6.

———. 1993. Adult years bring new afflictions for DES "babies." *New York Times*, 10 February, 12.

Brown, D. J. J. 1992. Spiralling connubia in the highlands of New Guinea. *Man* 27, no. 4:821–42.

Brownlee, S. 1990. The body at war: Baring the secrets of the immune system. *U.S. News and World Report*, 2 July, 48–54.

Burgess, J., M. Marten, and R. Taylor. 1987 *Microcosmos*. Cambridge: Cambridge University Press.

Burkard, W. E., R. L. Chambers, and F. W. Maroney. 1950. *Good health is fun*. Chicago: Lyons & Carnahan.

Burnet, F. M. 1962. *The integrity of the body: A discussion of modern immunological ideas*. Cambridge, Mass.: Harvard University Press.

Bylinsky, G. 1992. New weapons against AIDS. *Fortune*, 30 November, 104–7.

Byrne, J. A. 1993. Reengineering: Beyond the buzzword. *Business Week*, 24 May, 12.

Callon, M. 1986. Some elements of a sociology of translation: Domestication of the scallops and the fishermen of St. Brieuc Bay. In *Power, action and belief*, ed. J. Law. London: Routledge & Kegan Paul.

Cambrosio, A., and P. Keating. 1992. A Matter of FACS: Constituting novel entities in immunology. *Medical Anthropology Quarterly* 6, no. 4:362–84.

Campion, E. W. 1993. Why unconventional medicine? *New England Journal of Medicine* 328, no. 4 (28 January): 282–83.

Cancer and seasons. 1992. *New York Times*, 26 May, 8.

Canguilhem, G. [1977] 1988. *Ideology and rationality in the history of the life sciences*. Translated by Arthur Goldhammer. Cambridge, Mass.: MIT Press.

Cantor, N., and J. F. Kihlstrom. 1987. *Personality and social intelligence*. Englewood Cliffs, N.J.: Prentice-Hall.

Carton, B. 1993. Jerome Groopman, AIDS warrior. *Boston Globe*, 24 June, 53.

Change at the top for the F.B.I. 1993. *New York Times*, 21 July, A14. Editorial.

Chapman, G. 1992. Push comes to shove on technology policy. *Technology Review* 95, no. 8 (November): 42–49.

Charlesworth, M., L. Farrall, T. Stokes, and D. Turnbull. 1989. *Life among the scientists: An anthropological study of an Australian scientific community*. Melbourne: Oxford University Press.

Chase, M. 1992. AIDS meeting is dominated by reports of disease in HIV-negative patients. *Wall Street Journal*, 24 July, 4.

Cheater, A. 1993. Globalization and the new technologies of knowing: Anthropological calculus or chaos? Opening address to the fourth decennial conference of the Association of Social Anthropologists of the Commonwealth, Oxford, July.

Cherry, D. 1988. AIDS virus. In *Risky business*, ed. S. A. Winterhalter. San Francisco: San Francisco AIDS Foundation.

Chopra, D. 1989. *Quantum healing: Exploring the frontiers of mind/body medicine*. New York: Bantam.

Cimons, M. 1992. Possibility of new virus dominates AIDS conference. *Los Angeles Times*, 25 July, 6.

Claeson, B., E. Martin, W. Richardson, M. Schoch-Spana, and K. Taussig. 1991. "Scientific literacy": What it is, why it's important, and why scientists think we don't have it: The case of immunology and the immune system. Typescript.

Clark, K. 1993. 21,200 jobs lost in Md. last year. *Baltimore Sun*, 27 April, 1.

Clark, R. L., and R. W. Cumley. 1953. *The book of health*. Houston: Elsevier.

Clarke, A. E. 1987. Research materials and reproductive science in the United States, 1910–1940. In *Physiology in the American context, 1850–1940*, ed. G. L. Geison. Baltimore: Williams & Wilkins.

Clayton, J., and S. Campbell. 1992. How Baltimore stacks up. *Baltimore Magazine*, May, 34–39, 70.

Clendening, L. 1930. *The human body*. Garden City, N.Y.: Garden City.

Clerc, G. 1991. Artherosclerosis as an immune disease? *Medical Hypotheses* 36, no. 1 (September): 24–26.

Cocaine and immunity. 1988. *American Family Physician* 37, no. 6 (June): 322.

Cohen, I. R. 1987. The self, the world and autoimmunity. *Scientific American* 258, no. 4:52–60.

Cohen, J. 1992. AIDS research shifts to immunity. *Science* 257 (10 July): 152–54.

Conkin, D. 1992. Anthropologists talk about AIDS, enrage colleagues. *Bay Area Reporter*, 10 December, 5.

Connor, S. 1989. *Postmodernist culture: An introduction to theories of the contemporary*. Oxford: Blackwell.

Copeland, B. 1992. Review of *The immune system: Our internal defender*. *Book Report* 11:64.

Coppa, D. F. 1993. Chaos theory suggests a new paradigm for nursing science. *Journal of Advanced Nursing* 18, no. 6 (June): 985–91.

Corporate trainers manage to keep jobs. 1992. *Baltimore Sun*, 28 August, 1.

Corrigan, P. 1988. "Innocent stupidities": De-picturing (human) nature: On hopeful resistances and possible refusals: Celebrating difference(s) — again. In *Picturing power: Visual depiction and social relations*, ed. G. Fyfe and J. Law (*Sociological Review* Monograph no. 35). London: Routledge.

Coughlan, R. 1955. Science moves in on viruses. *Life*, 20 June, 122–36.

Coughlin, E. K. 1992. Tempers flare over AIDS session at anthropologists' annual meeting. *Chronicle of Higher Education*, 16 December, A8.

Cournoyer, C. 1991. *What about immunizations?* Santa Cruz, Calif.: Nelson's.

Coutinho, L., D. Forni, D. Holmberg, F. Ivars, and N. Vaz. 1984. From an antigen-centered, clonal perspective of immune responses to an organism-centered, network perspective of autonomous activity in a self-referential immune system. *Immunological Reviews* 79:151–68.

Crawford, R. 1980. Healthism and the medicalization of everyday life. *International Journal of Health Services* 10, no. 3:365–88.

Creedon, J. 1992. Second opinions on AIDS. *Utne Reader*, no. 53 (September/October): 17–18.

Crichton, M. 1990. *Jurassic Park: A novel*. New York: Knopf.

Crosby, P. B. 1984. *Quality without tears: The art of hassle-free management*. New York: McGraw-Hill.

Csikszentmihalyi, M. 1990. *Flow: The psychology of optimal experience*. New York: Harper & Row.

Csikszentmihalyi, M., and I. S. Csikszentmihalyi. 1990. Adventure and the flow experience. In *Adventure education*, ed. J. C. Miles and S. Priest. State College, Pa.: Venture.

Davis, W. J. 1989. Allergies: Introduction. In *Columbia University College of Physicians and Surgeons Complete home medical guide*, vol. 2. New York: Crown.

Deal, T. E., and A. A. Kennedy. 1982. *Corporate cultures: The rites and rituals of corporate life*. Reading, Mass.: Addison-Wesley.

A decoy for AIDS? 1988. *Economist*, 16 January, 81.

The defenders: Stop the invasion of the beauty snatchers. 1987. *Mademoiselle*, August, 222.

Defending children from disease. 1979. *Christian Science Monitor*, 4 September, 25.

Degler, C. N. 1991. *In search of human nature: The decline and revival of Darwinism in American social thought*. New York: Oxford University Press.

deLange, P. 1991. Move it! Regular exercise can improve the function of the immune system and may help lower the risk of cancer. *Vibrant Life* 7 (May): 10–13.

DeLillo, D. 1984. *White noise*. New York: Penguin.

Deming, W. E. 1993. *The new economics: For industry, government, education*. Cambridge, Mass.: MIT Center for Advanced Engineering Study.

DeParle, J. 1993. With shots, it's not only about costs, but stories. *New York Times*, 16 May, 1.

DeSchepper, L. 1989. *Peak immunity: How to fight Epstein-Barr virus, candida, herpes simplex and other immuno-depressive disorders and win*. Santa Monica, Calif.: Luc DeSchepper.

Diamond, J. 1992. The arrow of disease. *Discover* 13, no. 10 (October): 64–73.

Diekstra, R. 1988. Building defence. *World Health*, November, 28–29.

Diet and fitness: Five immune boosting eats. 1993. *Young Miss*, February, 70.

DiGiacomo, S. H. 1992. Metaphor as illness: Postmodern dilemmas in the representation of body, mind and disorder. *Medical Anthropology* 14:109–37.

Divorce and illness. 1987. *New York Times*, 24 February, 6.

Douglas, M. 1985. *Risk acceptability according to the social sciences*. New York: Russell Sage.

Dreher, H. 1992. The healing power of confession. *Natural Health*, July, 74–80.

Drucker, P. F. 1989. *The new realities*. New York: Harper & Row.

———. 1992. *Managing for the future: The 1990s and beyond*. New York: Penguin.

———. 1993. *Post-capitalist society*. New York: HarperCollins.

Duesberg, P. H. 1988. HIV is not the cause of AIDS. *Science* 241:514–16.

———. 1991. AIDS epidemiology: inconsistencies with human immunodeficiency virus and with infectious disease. *Proceedings of the National Academy of Sciences of the United States of America* 88, no. 4 (15 February): 1575–79.

Duggan, R. M. 1993. *Alternative medicine gets a hearing at the White House*. Columbia, Md.: Traditional Acupuncture Institute.

Dumaine, B. 1992. Is big still good? *Fortune*, 20 April, 50–60.

Duster, T. 1990. *Backdoor to eugenics*. London: Routledge.

Dwyer, J. M. 1988. *The body at war: The miracle of the immune system*. New York: New American Library.

Edelman, G. M. 1975. The shock of molecular recognition. In *Molecular Approaches to Immunology*, ed. E. E. Smith and D. W. Ribbons. New York: Academic.

———. 1987. *Neural Darwinism: The theory of neuronal group selection*. New York: Basic.

———. 1992. *Bright air, brilliant fire: On the matter of the mind*. New York: Basic.

Edidin, M. 1991. The biology of immune responses. In *The great ideas today*, 1991. Chicago: Encyclopedia Britannica.

Eisenberg, D. M., et al. 1993. Unconventional medicine in the United States: Prevalence, costs, and patterns of use. *New England Journal of Medicine* 328, no. 4:246–52.

Elliott, S. 1989. ABCs of immunology. *Healthsharing* 10, no. 2:17–19.

Ellis, R. W., ed. 1992. *Vaccines: New approaches to immunological problems*. Boston: Butterworth-Heinemann.

Endroczi, E. 1989. Recent development in hormone research. *Acta Physiologica Hungarica* 73, no. 4:417–32.

Engel, G. L. 1977. The need for a new medical model: A challenge for biomedicine. *Science* 196, no. 4286 (8 April): 129–36.

Engel, L. 1955. Battle of the labs. *New York Times Magazine*, 27 March, 63–65.

Euler, L. [1736] 1912. Mechanica sive motus scientia analytice exposita. In *Opera omnia*, 2d ser., vol. 1. Leipzig: Teubneri.

Fee, E., and D. M. Fox, eds. 1992. *AIDS: The making of a chronic disease*. Berkeley and Los Angeles: University of California Press.

Fee, E., and D. Porter. 1992. Public health, preventive medicine and professionalization: England and America in the nineteenth century. In *Medicine in society: Historical essays*, ed. A. Wear. Cambridge: Cambridge University Press.

Fee, E., L. Shopes, and L. Zeidman, eds. 1991. *The Baltimore book*. Philadelphia: Temple University Press.

Ferguson, K. E. 1984. *The feminist case against bureaucracy*. Philadelphia: Temple University Press.

Field, N. 1991. *In the realm of a dying emperor*. New York: Pantheon.

Fisher, L. M. 1991. Sneaking past the immune system to deliver toxic drugs to tumors. *New York Times*, 23 October, 5.

Fiske, J. 1987. *Television culture*. London: Routledge.

Five Texas girls say they had sex with an HIV-infected male to get into gang. 1993. *Baltimore Sun*, 27 April, 7.

Flanagan, B. 1993. Architect to client: "Let's work together." *New York Times*, 13 May, 1.

Flaste, R., ed. 1991. *The New York Times book of science literacy: What everyone needs to know from Newton to the knuckleball.* New York: Times Books.

Fleck, L. [1935] 1979. *Genesis and development of a scientific fact.* Chicago: University of Chicago Press.

Folkers, G. 1993. Maternal immunization: Vaccinating mom to protect baby, too. *Dateline: NIAID*, June, 1, 3, 5, 12.

Follett, M. P. 1918. *The new state: Group organization and the solution of popular government.* New York: Longmans, Green.

Foreman, J. 1992. Scientists predicting declining barriers to human longevity — to age 200 or more. *Baltimore Sun*, 10 October, 1.

Foucault, M. 1979. *Discipline and punish: The birth of the prison.* New York: Vintage.

———. 1980. *Power/knowledge: Selected interviews and other writings, 1972–1977.* New York: Pantheon.

———. 1991. Questions of method. In *The Foucault Effect: Studies in governmentality*, ed. G. Burchell, C. Gordon, and P. Miller. Chicago: University of Chicago Press.

Fox, A., and B. Fox. 1990. *Immune for life: Live longer and better by strengthening your doctor within.* Rocklin, Calif.: Prima.

Freeman, R. B. 1993. How much has de-unionization contributed to the rise in male earnings inequality? In *Uneven tides: Rising inequality in America*, ed. S. Danziger and P. Gottschalk. New York: Russell Sage.

Fumento, M. 1992. A complicated disease won't have simple answers. *Los Angeles Times*, 28 July, 7.

Gagnon, J. H. 1992. Epidemics and researchers: AIDS and the practice of social studies. In *The time of AIDS: Social analysis, theory, and method*, ed. S. Lindenbaum and G. Herdt. Newbury Park, Calif.: Sage.

Galland, L. 1988. *Superimmunity for kids.* New York: Dell.

Gane, M. 1991. *Baudrillard: Critical and fatal theory.* London: Routledge.

Garrahan, P., and P. Stewart. 1993. Working for Nissan. *Science as Culture* 3, no. 3:319–45.

Gates, J. 1989. Aging and the immune system. *Vibrant Life* 5 (September): 16–20.

Geertz, C. 1983a. Common sense as a cultural system. In *Local knowledge: Further essays in interpretive anthropology.* New York: Basic.

———. 1983b. Found in translation: On the social history of the moral imagination. In *Local knowledge: Further essays in interpretive anthropology.* New York: Basic.

Gelderman, C. 1981. *Henry Ford: The wayward capitalist.* New York: St. Martin's.

Gelman, R. G. 1992. *Body battles*. New York: Scholastic.

Gergen, K. J. 1991. *The saturated self: Dilemmas of identity in contemporary life*. New York: Basic.

Gerstenzang, J. 1993. AIDS to have little impact on society, study says. *Baltimore Sun,* 5 February, 1, 13.

Gilbert, S. 1992. Harnessing the power of light. *New York Times Magazine*, 26 April, 16–28.

Gilbreth, F. B., and E. G. Carey. 1948. *Cheaper by the dozen*. New York: Bantam.

Gitlin, T., ed. 1987. *Watching television*. New York: Pantheon.

Gladwell, M. 1992a. Meeting shows wide gap in knowledge about AIDS. *Washington Post*, 26 July, 26.

———. 1992b. Officials respond cautiously to reports of mysterious AIDS-like disease. *Washington Post*, 22 July, 4.

Glass, M. W., A. M. Schultz, B. J. Mathieson, D. Lawrence, S. Wescott, and W. C. Koff. 1990. Second Annual Meeting of the National Cooperative Vaccine Development Groups for AIDS. 15–18 October 1989; Fort Lauderdale, Florida. *Vaccine* 8, no. 4 (August): 413–14.

Gleick, J. 1987. *Chaos: Making a new science*. New York: Penguin.

Goffman, E. 1959. *The presentation of self in everyday life*. New York: Anchor.

Goldstein, A. 1992. Stung by criticism, Magic re-retires. *Baltimore Sun*, 3 November, 1, 2.

Goldstein, R. 1991. The implicated and the immune: Responses to AIDS in the arts and popular culture. In *A disease of society: Cultural and institutional responses to AIDS*, ed. D. Nelkin, D. P. Willis, and S. V. Parris. Cambridge: Cambridge University Press.

Goleman, D. 1985. Strong emotional response to disease may bolster patient's immune system. *New York Times*, 22 October, 1–2.

———. 1989. Researchers find that optimism helps the body's defense system. *New York Times*, 20 April, 9.

———. 1990. Support groups may do more in cancer than relieve the mind. *New York Times*, 18 October, 8.

———. 1992. New light on how stress erodes health. *New York Times*, 15 December, 1.

Gorman, C. 1992. Invincible AIDS. *Time*, 3 August, 26–30.

Gould, S. J. 1989. *Wonderful life: The Burgess Shale and the nature of history*. New York: Norton.

———. 1993. Dinomania. *New York Review of Books*, 12 August, 51–56.

Grady, D. 1992. Think right, stay well? (Can the mind improve the immune system?). *American Health* 11, no. 9 (November): 50–54.

Graeub, R. 1992. *The Petkau effect: Nuclear radiation, people and trees*. New York: Four Walls Eight Windows.

Gramich, E. M., R. Kasten, and F. Sammartino. 1993. Growing inequality in the 1980s: The role of federal taxes and cash transfers. In *Uneven tides: Rising inequality in America*, ed. S. Danziger and P. Gottschalk. New York: Russell Sage.

Gramsci, A. 1971. Americanism and Fordism. In *Selections from the prison notebooks of Antonio Gramsci*, ed. Q. Hoare and G. N. Smith. New York: International Publishers.

Greene, J. H., and D. Thompson. 1990. Outward bound USA. In *Adventure education*, ed. J. C. Miles and S. Priest. State College, Pa.: Venture.

Grmek, M. D. 1990. *History of AIDS: Emergence and origin of a modern pandemic*. Princeton, N.J.: Princeton University Press.

Gross, M. Z. 1949. Are we getting anywhere with polio. *Better Homes and Gardens*, August, 29, 130–31.

Guillory, J. 1993. *Cultural capital: The problem of literary canon formation*. Chicago: University of Chicago Press.

Gusterson, H. 1991. Nuclear war, the Gulf War, and the disappearing body. *Journal of Urban and Cultural Studies* 2, no. 1:45–55.

Halperin, R. 1990. *The livelihood of kin: Making ends meet "the Kentucky way."* Austin: University of Texas Press.

Hammer, M., and J. Champy. 1993. *Reengineering the corporation: A manifesto for business revolution*. New York: HarperCollins.

Haraway, D. 1989. *Primate visions: Gender, race, and nature in the world of modern science*. New York: Routledge.

———. 1991. The politics of postmodern bodies: Constitutions of self in immune system discourse. In *Simians, cyborgs, and women*. New York: Routledge.

Harvey, D. 1989. *The condition of postmodernity: An enquiry into the origins of social change*. Oxford: Blackwell.

———. 1991a. Flexibility: Threat or opportunity? *Socialist Review* 21, no. 1:65–77.

———. 1991b. A view from Federal Hill. In *The Baltimore book*, ed. E. Fee, L. Shopes, and L. Zeidman. Philadelphia: Temple University Press.

Have you a health conscience? 1952. *Today's Health* 13 (October): 70–71.

Hayles, N. K. 1990. *Chaos bound: Orderly disorder in contemporary literature and science*. Ithaca, N.Y.: Cornell University Press.

Hazen, R. M., and J. Trefil. 1991a. Quick? What's a quark? *New York Times Magazine*, 13 January, 26.

———. 1991b. *Science matters: Achieving scientific literacy*. New York: Doubleday.

Heale, M. J. 1990. *American anti-communism: Combating the enemy within, 1830–1970*. Baltimore: Johns Hopkins University Press.

Heimoff, S. 1992. Test ideas with science, not scorn. *Los Angeles Times*, 23 July, 7.

Heller, L. 1988. Beulah, peel me a persimmon. *GQ*, October, 211–14.

Helmreich, S. 1992. Computer viruses, human bodies, and the logic of the nation state in the age of flexible specialization. Typescript.

Help may be too late for Somalis on brink. 1992. *Baltimore Sun*, 7 December, 4.

Help prevent infantile paralysis. 1948. *House Beautiful*, July, 89.

Henig, R. M. 1992. Flu pandemic. *New York Times*, 29 November, 28–31, 55, 64, 66–67.

Hess, D. J. 1992. Introduction: The new ethnography and the anthropology of science and technology. In *Knowledge and society: The anthropology of science and technology*, ed. D. J. Hess and L. L. Layne, Knowledge and Society 9, ed. A. Ripp. Greenwich, Conn.: JAI.

———. 1993. *Science in the new age: The paranormal, its defenders and debunkers, and American culture*. Madison: University of Wisconsin Press.

Hesse, M. B. 1961. *Forces and fields: The concept of action at a distance in the history of physics*. London: Nelson & Sons.

Hiam, A. 1990. *The vest-pocket CEO: Decision-making tools for executives*. Englewood Cliffs, N.J.: Prentice-Hall.

———. 1992. *Closing the quality gap: Lessons from America's leading companies*. Englewood Cliffs, N.J.: Prentice-Hall.

Hilts, P. J. 1992. F.D.A. acts to halt breast implants made of silicone. *New York Times*, 7 January, 1.

Hindley, J., and C. King. 1975. *How your body works*. London: Usborne.

Hobbs, C., and D. DeSilver. 1989. A new strategy for rebuilding immunity. *Vegetarian Times*, November, 72–77.

Hofstadter, R. [1955] 1992. *Social Darwinism in American thought*. Boston: Beacon.

Holtzman, N. A. 1989. *Proceed with caution: Predicting genetic risks in the recombinant DNA era*. Baltimore: Johns Hopkins University Press.

Hoppa, J. 1993. Temporaries have to do without a safety net. *New York Times*, 21 July, 16.

Horwitz, T. 1992. Lethal cuisine takes high toll in Glasgow, West's sickest city. *Wall Street Journal*, 22 September, 1, 12.

Howe, H. A. 1951a. Can we vaccinate against polio? *Harpers*, April, 37–42.

———. 1951b. Those virus diseases. *Harpers*, March, 34–38.

Hubbard, R., and E. Wald. 1993. *Exploding the gene myth: How genetic information is produced and manipulated by scientists, physicians, employers, insurance companies, educators, and law enforcers.* Boston: Beacon.

Hunt, J. S. 1990. Philosophy of adventure education. In *Adventure education*, ed. J. C. Miles and S. Priest. State College, Pa.: Venture.

Immunex advances in bid for easing transplants. 1990. *New York Times*, 11 May, 2.

Irigaray, L. 1993. *Je, tu, nous: Toward a culture of difference.* New York: Routledge.

Jackson, K. T. 1985. *Crabgrass frontier: The suburbanization of the United States.* New York: Oxford University Press.

Jameson, F. 1984. Postmodernism, or the cultural logic of late capitalism. *New Left Review*, 146:52–92.

Janković, B. D. 1989. The relationship between the immune system and the nervous system: Old and new strategies. In *Immunology, 1930–80*: Essays on the History of Immunology, ed. P. M. H. Mazumdar. Toronto: Wall & Thompson.

Jaret, P. 1986. Our immune system: The wars within. *National Geographic*, June, 702–35.

———. 1987. The wars within us. *Reader's Digest*, January, 164–76.

Jaroff, L. 1988. Stop that germ! *Time*, 23 May, 56–64.

Jemmott, J. B., and K. Magloire. 1988. Academic stress, social support, and secretory immunoglobulin A. *Journal of Personality and Social Psychology* 55, no. 5:803–10.

Jerne, N. K. 1974. Towards a network theory of the immune system. *Annals of the Pasteur Institute in Immunology* 125C:373–89.

Jewler, D. 1989. Diabetes and the immune system. *Diabetes Forecast* 42, no. 8 (August): 32–40.

JM. 1991. Autoimmunity explored in AIDS pathology. *Science*, 8 November, 799.

Johnson, S. J. 1987. *Going out of our minds: The metaphysics of liberation.* Freedom, Calif.: Crossing.

Jonsen, A. R., and J. Stryker, eds. 1993. *The social impact of AIDS in the United States.* Washington, D.C.: National Academy Press.

Juran, J. M. 1988. *Juran on planning for quality.* New York: Free Press.

Kantor, R. M. 1989. *When giants learn to dance.* New York: Simon & Schuster.

Karush, F. 1989. Metaphors in immunology. In *Immunology, 1930–80: Essays on the history of immunology*, ed. P. M. H. Mazumdar. Toronto: Wall & Thompson.

Kash, D. E. 1989. *Perpetual innovation: The new world of competition.* New York: Basic.

Keeping breast milk safe. 1989. *American Health* 8, no. 1 (January): 20–22.

Keller, E. F. 1985. *Reflections on gender and science*. New Haven, Conn.: Yale University Press.

———. 1992. *Secrets of life: Essays on language, gender and science*. New York: Routledge.

Keller, E. F., and C. R. Grontkowski. 1983. The mind's eye. In *Discovering Reality*, ed. S. Harding and M. B. Hintikka. Dordrecht: Reidel.

Kellert, S. H. 1993. *In the wake of chaos: Unpredictable order in dynamical systems*. Chicago: University of Chicago Press.

Kelly, K. 1991. Designing perpetual novelty: Selected notes from the second artificial life conference. In *Doing science*, ed. J. Brockman. New York: Prentice-Hall.

Keyes, K. 1982. *The hundredth monkey*. Coos Bay, Oreg.: Vision.

Kimball, J. W. 1986. *Introduction to immunology*. New York: Macmillan.

Kimber, D. C., C. E. Gray, and C. E. Stackpole. 1934. *Textbook of anatomy and physiology*. New York: Macmillan.

Knorr-Cetina, K. 1981. *The manufacture of knowledge: An essay on the constructivist and contextual nature of science*. Oxford: Pergamon.

———. 1983. The ethnographic study of scientific work: Towards a constructivist interpretation of science. In *Science observed: Perspectives on the social study of science*, ed. K. Knorr-Cetina and M. Mulkay. London: Sage.

Kolata, G. 1988. New research yields clues in fight against autoimmune diseases. *New York Times*, 19 January, 3.

———. 1992. Immune cells are taught to kill a virus; cells might be trained to attack AIDS or cancer. *New York Times*, 10 July, 12, 15.

———. 1993. Nerve cells tied to immune system. *New York Times*, 13 May, 12.

Kramer, L. 1992. Name an AIDS high command. *New York Times*, 15 November, 19.

Kreisler, K. von. 1993. The healing powers of sex. *Reader's Digest*, June, 17–20.

Laabs, J. J. 1991. Team training goes outdoors. *Personnel Journal* 70, no. 6:56–63.

LaForge, R. 1989. Does fitness strengthen the immune system? *Executive Health Report* 26 (December):6–7.

Laliberte, R. 1992. The best defense. *Men's Health*, September, 56–60.

Lang, S. S. 1988. Can workouts prevent illness? *Vogue*, September, 510.

Langfitt, F. 1993. Access "the world" via Seymour. *Baltimore Sun*, 1 November, 1A, 4A.

Larsen, R. A. 1985. "You are feeling very healthy. . . . " *Health*, June, 21.

Latour, B. 1983. Give me a laboratory and I will raise the world. In *Science observed: Perspectives on the social study of science*, ed. K. D. Knorr-Cetina and M. Mulkay. London: Sage.

———. 1986. Visualization and cognition: Thinking with eyes and hands. *Knowledge and Society: Studies in the Sociology of Culture Past and Present* 6:1–40.

———. 1987. *Science in action*. Cambridge, Mass.: Harvard University Press.

———. 1988. *The pasteurization of France*. Cambridge, Mass.: Harvard University Press.

———. 1990. Postmodern? No, simply *amodern!* Steps towards an anthropology of science. *Studies in the History and Philosophy of Science* 21, no. 1:145–71.

Latour, B., and S. Woolgar. 1986. *Laboratory life: The construction of scientific facts*. Princeton, N.J.: Princeton University Press.

Lave, J. 1986. The values of quantification. In *Power, action and belief*, ed. J. Law. London: Routledge & Kegan Paul.

———. 1988. *Cognition in practice: Mind, mathematics, and culture in everyday life*. Cambridge: Cambridge University Press.

Lear, M. W. 1993. She's no jockette. *New York Times Magazine*, 25 July, 20–52.

Leavitt, J. W. 1992. "Typhoid Mary" strikes back: Bacteriological theory and practice in early twentieth-century public health. *Isis* 83:608–29.

Levin, D. M., and G. F. Solomon. 1990. The discursive formation of the body in the history of medicine. *Journal of Medicine and Philosophy* 15, no. 5:515–37.

Lewis, J. R., and J. G. Melton. 1992. *Perspectives on the new age*. Albany: State University of New York Press.

Lewontin, R. C. 1991. *Biology as ideology: The doctrine of DNA*. New York: HarperCollins.

Lewthwaite, G. A. 1993. The shrinking workplace. *Baltimore Sun*, 25 July, 1, 8A.

Libby, P., and G. K. Hansson. 1991. Involvement of the immune system in human atherogenesis: Current knowledge and unanswered questions. *Laboratory Investigation* 64, no. 1:5–15.

Libby, P., R. N. Salomon, D. D. Payne, F. J. Schoen, and J. S. Pober. 1989. Functions of vascular wall cells related to development of transplantation-associated coronary arteriosclerosis. *Transplantation Proceedings* 21, no. 4 (August): 3677–84.

Linton, R. 1936. *The study of man: An introduction*. New York: Appleton-Century.

Lobsenz, A. 1954. Do you know what's good for you? *Woman's Home Companion*, December, 54, 88.

Loynes, C. 1990. Development training in the United Kingdom. In *Adventure education*, ed. J. C. Miles and S. Priest. State College, Pa.: Venture.

Luks, A. 1991. *The healing power of doing good: The health and spiritual benefits of helping others*. New York: Fawcett Columbine.

Lynch, M. 1985. *Art and artifact in laboratory science: A study of shop work and shop talk in a research laboratory*. London: Routledge & Kegan Paul.

McAvoy, L. 1990. Rescue-free wilderness areas. In *Adventure education*, ed. J. C. Miles and S. Priest. State College, Pa.: Venture.

McCaleb, R. 1990. Astragalus: Immunity enhancer. *Better Nutrition for Today's Living* 52 (October): 22–25.

McGuire, M. B. 1988. *Ritual healing in suburban America*. New Brunswick, N.J.: Rutgers University Press.

Mah, H. 1991. Suppressing the text: The metaphysics of ethnographic history in Darnton's great cat massacre. *History Workshop Journal* 31:1–20.

Maier, S. F., and M. Laudenslager. 1985. Stress and health: Exploring the links. *Psychology Today*, August, 44–49.

Mann, J. 1992. Opening remarks. In *Conference summary report: VIII International Conference on AIDS, III STD World Congress, Amsterdam, the Netherlands*. Cambridge, Mass.: Harvard AIDS Institute.

Markoff, J. 1992. Computer viruses: Just uncommon colds after all? *New York Times*, 1 November, 9.

Markus, G. 1987. Why is there no hermeneutics of natural sciences? Some preliminary theses. *Science in Context* 1, no. 1:5–51.

Mars, B. 1992. Natural remedies for a healthy immune system. Boulder, Colo.: Sounds True. Audiotape.

Marshall, W., and M. Schram, eds. 1993. *Mandate for change*. New York: Berkley.

Martin, E. 1992. The end of the body? *American Ethnologist* 19, no. 1:120–38.

Martin, E., L. Oaks, K. Taussig, and A. van der Straten. In press. AIDS, knowledge and discrimination in the inner city: An anthropological analysis of the experiences of injection drug users. In *Cyborgs and citadels: Anthropological interventions in technohuman practices*, ed. G. Downey, J. Dumit, and S. Traweek. Santa Fe, N.M.: School of American Research.

Martin, W. 1991. *Cape Cod*. New York: Warner.

Marx, K. [1859] 1970. *Contribution to the critique of political economy*. London: Lawrence & Wishart.

Maté, G. 1993. Why does the body sometimes declare war on itself? *Toronto Globe and Mail*, 14 June, 16.

Mathews, J. 1992. The cost of quality. *Newsweek*, 7 September, 48–49.

May, E. T. 1988. *Homeward bound: American families in the cold war era*. New York: Basic.

Mazumdar, P. M. H. 1975. The purpose of immunity: Landsteiner's interpretation of the human isoantibodies. *Journal of the History of Biology* 8, no. 1 (March): 115–33.

Merl, J. 1991. Schools to send layoff notices for "flexibility." *Los Angeles Times*, 5 March, 1.

Meyers, E. M. 1986. *Rebuilding America's cities: A policy analysis of the U.S. Conference of Mayors*. Cambridge, Mass.: Ballinger.

Michaud, E., and A. Feinstein. 1989. *Fighting disease: The complete guide to natural immune power*. Emmaus, Pa.: Rodale.

Miller, B. F., and R. Goode. 1960. *Man and his body*. New York: Simon & Schuster.

Miner, J. L. 1990. The creation of outward bound. In *Adventure education*, ed. J. C. Miles and S. Priest. State College, Pa.: Venture.

Mizel, S. B., and P. Jaret. 1985. *In self defense*. San Diego, Calif.: Harcourt Brace Jovanovich.

Moberg, C. L., and Z. A. Cohn, eds. 1990. *Launching the antibiotic era: Personal accounts of the discovery and use of the first antibiotics*. New York: Rockefeller University Press.

Modleski, T. 1991. *Feminism without women: Culture and criticism in a "postfeminist" age*. New York: Routledge.

Moffatt, A. S. 1988. Get a good night's rest. *American Health*, July, 54.

Molnar, M., and J. E. Skinner. 1992. Low-dimensional chaos in event-related brain potentials. *International Journal of Neuroscience* 66, nos. 3–4 (October): 263–76

Morley, D. 1992. *Television, audiences and cultural studies*. London: Routledge.

Morley, J. E., et al. 1987. Neuropeptides: Conductors of the immune orchestra. *Life Sciences* 41, no. 5:527–44.

Moulin, A. 1989. Immunology old and new: The beginning and the end. In *Immunology, 1930–80: Essays on the history of immunology*, ed. P. M. H. Mazumdar. Toronto: Wall & Thompson.

———. 1991. *Le dernier langage de la medécine: Histoire de l'immunologie de Pasteur au Sida*. Paris: Presses Universitaires de France.

Moyers, B. 1993. *Healing and the mind*. New York: Doubleday.

Munro-Faure, L., and M. Munro-Faure. 1992. *Implementing total quality management*. London: Pitman.

Muramoto, N. B. 1988. *Natural immunity: Insights on diet and AIDS*. Oroville, Calif.: George Ohsawa Macrobiotic Foundation.

Murphy, M. 1992. *The future of the body: Explorations into the further evolution of human nature*. Los Angeles: Tarcher.

Murray, F. 1990. Garlic offers exciting new benefits. *Better Nutrition for Today's Living*, December, 12–14.

Nader, L. 1990. *Harmony ideology: Justice and control in a Zapotec mountain village*. Stanford, Calif.: Stanford University Press.

Napier, A. D. 1992. *Foreign bodies: Performance, art, and symbolic anthropology*. Berkeley and Los Angeles: University of California Press.

National Institute of Allergy and Infectious Diseases. 1985. *Understanding the immune system*. Washington, D.C.

National Jewish Center for Immunology and Respiratory Medicine. 1989. *Immunology*. Washington, D.C.

Navarro, M. 1992. 68 U.S. patients in limbo: Caught in medical enigma. *New York Times*, 21 September, 1.

Neikirk, W. 1992. In Clinton's brave new world, jobs for the nimble. *Baltimore Sun*, 23 December, 13.

Networks: On a higher plane? 1991. *Immunology Today* 12, no. 5 (May): 154.

Nilsson, L. 1985. *The body victorious*. New York: Delacorte.

Nolan, P., and K. O'Donnell. 1991. Restructuring and the politics of industrial renewal: The limits of flexible specialization. In *Farewell to Flexibility?* ed. A. Pollert. Oxford: Blackwell.

Noyelle, T. J., and T. M. Stanback. 1984. *The economic transformation of American cities*. Totowa, N.J.: Rowman & Allanheld.

Obeyesekere, G. 1990. *The work of culture: Symbolic transformation in psychoanalysis and anthropology*. Chicago: University of Chicago Press.

O'Connor, B. 1949. The conquest of infantile paralysis. *Hygeia* 27 (June): 388–89, 428–30.

OED. 1989. *The Oxford English dictionary*. 2d ed. Oxford: Clarendon.

Oliver, J. L., P. Bernaola-Galvan, J. Guerrero-Garcia, and R. Roman-Roldan. 1993. Entropic profiles of DNA sequences through chaos-game-derived images. *Journal of Theoretical Biology* 160, no. 4 (February): 457–70.

Olson, S. H. 1980. *Baltimore: The building of an American city*. Baltimore: Johns Hopkins University Press.

O'Mara, P., ed. 1992. *Vaccinations: The rest of the story*. Santa Fe, N.M.: Mothering.

Ornstein, R., and D. Sobel. 1987. The healing brain. *Psychology Today*, March, 48–52.

Osborne, D., and T. Gaebler. 1992. *Reinventing government: How the entrepreneurial spirit is transforming the public sector*. Reading, Mass.: Addison-Wesley.

Ostreicher, D., and D. Klein. 1987. Maximize your immune system. *McCall's*, October, 79–80.

Page, J. 1981. *Blood: The river of life*. Washington, D.C.: U.S. News Books.

Pagels, H. R. 1989. *The dreams of reason: The computer and the rise of the sciences of complexity*. New York: Bantam.

Pain, R. 1991. Protein dynamics: A case of a flexible friend. *Nature* 354, no. 6352 (5 December): 353–54.

Palca, J. 1991. On the track of an elusive disease. *Science* 254, no. 5039 (20 December): 1726–28.

Patton, C. 1990. *Inventing AIDS*. New York: Routledge.

Patton, P. 1993. The virtual office becomes reality. *New York Times*, 28 October, C1, C6.

Peabody, J. E., and A. E. Hunt. 1934. *Biology and human welfare*. New York: Macmillan.

Pearsall, P. 1987. *Super immunity: Master your emotions and improve your health*. New York: Fawcett.

Perrow, C. 1984. *Normal accidents: Living with high risk technologies*. New York: Basic.

Pert, C. 1993. The chemical communicators. In *Healing and the mind*, ed. B. D. Moyers and B. S. Flowers. New York: Doubleday.

Petchesky, R. P. 1981. Antiabortion, antifeminism and the rise of the new Right. *Feminist Studies* 7, no. 2:206–46.

Peters, T. 1992. *Liberation management*. New York: Knopf.

Phenix, K. 1992. Educational software. *Wilson Library Bulletin* 66 (June): 90.

Piore, M. J., and C. F. Sabel. 1984. *The second industrial divide: Possibilities for prosperity*. New York: Basic.

Pollert, A. 1991. The orthodoxy of flexibility. In *Farewell to flexibility?* ed. A. Pollert. Oxford: Blackwell.

Pomeranz, H., and I. S. Koll. 1957. *The family physician*. New York: Greystone.

Port, O. 1992. Special report: Quality: Small and midsize companies seize the challenge — not a moment too soon. *Business Week*, 30 November, 66–75.

Potts, E., and M. Morra. 1986. *Understanding your immune system*. New York: Avon.

Preston, R. 1987. *First light: The search for the edge of the universe*. New York: Atlantic Monthly Press.

———. 1992. Crisis in the hot zone. *New Yorker*, 26 October, 58–81.

Price, R. 1992. *Clockers*. New York: Houghton Mifflin.

Rabinbach, A. 1990. *The human motor: Energy, fatigue, and the origins of modernity*. New York: Basic.

Rabinow, P. 1992a. Artificiality and enlightenment: From sociobiology to biosociality. In *Incorporations: Zone 6*, ed. J. Crary and S. Kwinter. New York: Urzone.

————. 1992b. Severing the ties: Fragmentation and redemption in late modernity. In *The anthropology of science and technology: Knowledge and society* 9, ed. D. Hess and L. Layne. Greenwich, Conn.: JAI.

Rapp, R. 1988. Chromosomes and communication: The discourse of genetic counseling. *Medical Anthropology Quarterly* 2, no.2:143–57.

Rasmussen, N. 1992. Saving the cell's power plant: The mitochondrion and biological electron microscopy in the 1950s. Paper presented at the Princeton "Visualization Workshop."

Ratcliff, J. D. 1947. The latest on polio. *Woman's Home Companion*, August, 34–35.

Reich, R. B. 1991. *The resurgent liberal (and other unfashionable prophecies)*. New York: Vintage.

————. 1992. *The work of nations*. New York: Vintage.

Rhinesmith, S. H. 1993. *A manager's guide to globalization: Six keys to success in a changing world*. Alexandria, Va.: American Society for Training and Development.

Richman, L. S. 1993. How to protect your financial future. *Fortune*, 25 January, 58–60.

Rifkin, J. 1983. *Algeny: A new word — a new world*. New York: Penguin.

Ritchie, J. W. 1918. *Primer of sanitation and physiology*. Yonkers-on-Hudson, N.Y.: World.

————. 1948. *Biology and human affairs*. Yonders-on-Hudson, N.Y.: World.

Robbins, B., ed. 1993. *The phantom public sphere*. Minneapolis: University of Minnesota Press.

Roberts, H. V., and B. F. Sergesketter. 1993. *Quality is personal: A foundation for total quality management*. New York: Free Press.

Roberts, M. 1987. Moody immunity. *Psychology Today*, November, 14.

Robertson, R. 1992. *Globalization: Social theory and global culture*. London: Sage.

Rogers, C. R. 1951. *Client-centered therapy: Its current practice, implications, and theory*. Boston: Houghton Mifflin.

Rogers, N. 1992. *Dirt and disease: Polio before FDR*. New Brunswick, N.J.: Rutgers University Press.

Root-Bernstein, R. S. 1992. AIDS is more than HIV: Part I. *Genetic Engineering News* 12, no. 13 (1 September): 4–6.

————. 1993. *Rethinking AIDS: The tragic cost of premature consensus.* New York: Free Press.

Rosenbaum, D. E. 1993. White House budget stand is denounced by Moynihan. *New York Times*, 24 July, 26.

Rosenberg, C. E. 1979a. Florence Nightingale on contagion: The hospital as moral universe. In *Healing and history: Essays for George Rosen*, ed. C. E. Rosenberg. New York: Science History.

————. 1979b. The therapeutic revolution: Medicine, meaning, and social change in nineteenth-century America. In *The therapeutic revolution: Essays in the social history of American medicine*, ed. M. J. Vogel and C. E. Rosenberg. Philadelphia: University of Pennsylvania Press.

————. 1983. Medical text and social context: Explaining William Buchan's "domestic medicine." *Bulletin of the History of Medicine*, 57:22–42.

————. 1989. Body and mind in nineteenth-century medicine: Some clinical origins of the neurosis construct. *Bulletin of the History of Medicine* 63, no. 2:185–97.

Rosenthal, E. 1989. Transplant patients illuminate link between cancer and immunity. *New York Times*, 5 December, 5.

————. 1993a. Doctors weigh the costs of a chicken pox vaccine. *New York Times*, 7 July, 1.

————. 1993b. Parents face questions on vaccinating infants for hepatitis B. *New York Times*, 3 March, 12.

Ross, A. 1991. *Strange weather: Culture, science and technology in the age of limits*. London: Verso.

Ross, R. 1990. Mechanisms of atherosclerosis — a review. *Advances in Nephrology from the Necker Hospital* 19:79–86.

————. 1993. The pathogenesis of atherosclerosis: A perspective for the 1990s. *Nature* 362, no. 6423 (29 April): 801–9.

Rouse, J. 1993. What are cultural studies of scientific knowledge? *Configurations* 1, no. 1:1–22.

Rouse, J. W. 1984. The case for vision. In *Rebuilding America's cities: Roads to recovery*, ed. P. R. Porter and D. C. Sweet. New Brunswick, N.J.: Center for Urban Policy Research.

Rubin, E. 1989. Review of *The immune system: Your magic doctor. School Library Journal* 35:58.

Rustin, M. 1989. The politics of post-Fordism; or, the trouble with "new times." *New Left Review* 175:54–77.

Sandoval, C. 1991. U.S. Third World feminism: The theory and method of oppositional consciousness in the postmodern world. *Genders* 10:1–24.

Sarris, M. 1992. Grim picture is painted for Md. economy. *Baltimore Sun*, 4 September, 1, 8.

Sawicki, J. 1991. *Disciplining Foucault: Feminism, power, and the body*. London: Routledge.

Scarry, E. 1985. *The body in pain: The making and unmaking of the world*. New York: Oxford University Press.

Schenker, I. 1988. The immune system approach in teaching AIDS to youngsters: Two unique programs for schools. In *The global impact of AIDS*, ed. A. F. Fleming, M. Carballo, D. W. FitzSimons, M. R. Bailey and J. Mann. New York: Liss.

———. 1992. *The immune system and AIDS: A multi-media health education program on AIDS prevention for schools*. Jerusalem: Jerusalem AIDS Project.

Schindler, L. W. 1988. *Understanding the immune system*. Washington, D.C.: U.S. Department of Health and Human Services.

Schmid, G. B. 1991. Chaos theory and schizophrenia: Elementary aspects. *Psychopathology* 24, no. 4:185–98.

Schriftgiesser, K. 1952. When 11 of 14 children were hit with polio. *Collier's*, November, 17–19.

Scott, J. W. 1992. Experience. In *Feminists theorize the political*, ed. J. Butler and J. W. Scott. New York: Routledge.

Sell, S. 1987. *Basic immunology: Immune mechanisms in health and disease*. New York: Elsevier.

Seltzer, M. 1992. *Bodies and machines*. New York: Routledge.

Senge, P. M. 1990. *The fifth discipline: The art and practice of the learning organization*. New York: Doubleday.

Sercarz, E. E., F. Celada, N. A. Mitchison, and T. Tada, eds. 1988. *The semiotics of cellular communication in the immune system*. Berlin: Springer.

Serinus, J., ed. 1987. *Psychoimmunity and the healing process*. Berkeley, Calif.: Celestial Arts.

Sewell, G., and B. Wilkinson. 1992. "Someone to watch over me": Surveillance, discipline and the just-in-time labour process. *Sociology: Journal of the British Sociological Association* 26, no. 2:271–89.

Sex is the best cure for a cold! 1993. *National Enquirer*, 9 March, 3.

Shapin, S. 1982. History of science and its sociological reconstructions. *History of Science* 20:157–211.

Shapin, S., and S. Schaffer. 1985. *Leviathan and the air-pump: Hobbes, Boyle, and the experimental life*. Princeton, N.J.: Princeton University Press.

Shapiro, S. 1993. "Ah, Zoh." *Baltimore Sun*, 18 April, 1.

Sheldrake, R. 1988. *The presence of the past: Morphic resonance and the habits of nature.* New York: Vintage.

———. 1991. *The rebirth of nature: The greening of science and God.* New York: Bantam.

Sherman, S. 1993. A brave new Darwinian workplace. *Fortune*, 25 January, 50–56.

Silverstein, A. M. 1989. *A history of immunology.* San Diego, Calif.: Academic.

Sinetar, M. 1991. *Developing a 21st century mind.* New York: Villard.

Skinner, J. E. 1993. Neurocardiology: Brain mechanisms underlying fatal cardiac arrhythmias. *Neurologic Clinics* 11, no. 2 (May): 325–51.

Smith, C. 1991. From 1960s' automation to flexible specialization: A *déjà vu* of technological panaceas. In *Farewell to flexibility?* ed. A. Pollert. London: Blackwell.

Solomon, G. F. 1987. Psychoneuroimmunology: Interactions between central nervous system and immune system. *Journal of Neuroscience Research* 18:1–9.

Solomon, G. F., D. Benton, J. E. Morley and L. Temoshok. 1989. Psychoimmune connections: Aging, immunity, health, and HIV infection. *Generations* 13:12–14.

Solomon, J. 1993. A touching presidency. *Newsweek*, 22 February, 44.

Sonnabend, J. A., S. S. Wittkin and D. T. Purtilo. 1984. A multifactorial model for the development of AIDS in homosexual men. *New York Academy of Science* 437:177.

Sontag, S. 1978. *Illness as metaphor.* New York: Ferrar, Straus, Giroux.

Spanbauer, S. 1993. Antivirus software: Search and destroy. *PC World*, May, 194–201.

Specter, M. 1992. Neglected for years, TB is back with strains that are deadlier (Tuberculosis: A killer returns, part 1). *New York Times*, 11 October, 1, 44.

Squire, S. 1987. New clues to the immune system. *New York Times*, 1 February, 32.

Stacey, R. 1992. *Managing chaos: Dynamic business strategies in an unpredictable world.* London: Kogan Page.

Stafford, B. 1991. *Body criticism: Imaging the unseen in Enlightenment art and medicine.* Cambridge, Mass.: MIT Press.

Star, S. L. 1991. Power, technologies and the phenomenology of conventions: On being allergic to onions. In *A sociology of monsters: Essays on power, technology and domination*, ed. J. Law. London: Routledge.

Starr, P. 1982. *The social transformation of American medicine.* New York: Basic.

Steinman, L. 1993. Autoimmune disease. *Scientific American* 269, no. 3 (September): 106–14.

Sterling, J. 1992. A new view of AIDS. *Genetic Engineering News* 12, no. 13 (1 September): 4.

Stevens, W. K. 1991. Balance of nature? What balance is that? *New York Times*, 22 October, 4.

Stevenson, L. G. 1955. Science down the drain: On the hostility of certain sanitarians to animal experimentation, bacteriology and immunology. *Bulletin of the History of Medicine* 29, no. 1 (January): 1–26.

Stolcke, V. 1992. The "right to difference" in an unequal world. Typescript.

———. 1993. Is sex to gender as race is to ethnicity? In *Gendered anthropology*, ed. T. del Valle. London: Routledge.

Strathern, M. In press. Nostalgia and the new genetics. In *The rhetoric of self-making*, ed. D. Battaglia. Berkeley and Los Angeles: University of California Press.

Sutphen, D. 1988. Strengthening your immune system: Subliminal programming with music. Malibu, Calif.: Valley of the Sun. Audiotape.

Terrace, V. 1985–86. *Encyclopedia of television series, pilots and specials.* 3 vols. New York: Zoetrope.

Thompson, L. 1989. A research gain for multiple sclerosis: New strategy that shuts down part of the immune system shows promise. *Washington Post*, 17 October, 7.

Three diseases pose deadliest risk to cats. 1992. In *Pet Media.* (Animal Health). Smith Kline Beecham brochure.

Tickner, L. 1988. *The spectacle of women: Imagery of the suffrage campaign.* Chicago: University of Chicago Press.

Tomes, N. 1990. The private side of public health: Sanitary science, domestic hygiene, and the germ theory, 1870–1900. *Bulletin of the History of Medicine* 64:509–39.

Total quality report card grades US firms. 1992. *AQP Report*, August, 1, 3.

Traweek, S. 1988. *Beamtimes and lifetimes: The world of high energy physics.* Cambridge, Mass.: Harvard University Press.

———. 1992. Border crossings: Narrative strategies in science studies and among physicists in Tsukuba Science City, Japan. In *Science as practice and culture*, ed. A. Pickering. Chicago: University of Chicago Press.

Treichler, P. A. 1987. AIDS, homophobia and biomedical discourse: An epidemic of signification. *Cultural Studies* 1, no. 3 (October): 263–305.

———. 1991. How to have theory in an epidemic: The evolution of AIDS treatment activism. In *Technoculture: Cultural Politics* 3, ed. C. Penley and A. Ross. Minneapolis: University of Minnesota Press.

———. 1992. AIDS, HIV, and the cultural construction of reality. In *The Time of AIDS: Social analysis, theory, and method*, ed. S. Lindenbaum and G. Herdt. Newbury Park, Calif.: Sage.

Truesdale, C. 1960. *The rational mechanics of flexible or elastic bodies, 1638–1788: Introduction to Leonhardi Euleri Opera omnia vol. X et XI seriei secundae*. Turici: Orell Füssli.

Tuchman, G. 1991. Pluralism and disdain: American culture today. In *America at century's end*, ed. A. Wolfe. Berkeley and Los Angeles: University of California Press.

Turkle, S. 1984. *The second self: Computers and the human spirit*. London: Granada.

Uexküll, T. von. 1988. Possible contribution of biosemiotics to the problem of communication among lymphocytes. In *The semiotics of cellular communication in the immune system*, ed. E. E. Sercarz, F. Celada, N. A. Mitchison, and T. Tada. Berlin: Springer.

Ungeheuer, F. 1992. The master detective, still on the case. *Time*, 3 August, 30.

Valentine, R. C. 1967. Electron microscopy of IgG immunoglobulins. In *Gamma globulins: Structure and control of biosynthesis: Proceedings of the Third Nobel Symposium, June 12–17, 1967, Stockholm*, ed. J. Killander. Stockholm: Almquist & Wiksell.

Varela, F. J., and A. Coutinho. 1991. Second generation immune networks. *Immunolody Today* 12, no. 5 (May): 159–66.

Vision of the future. 1954. *Time*, 1 November, 77–78.

Visions of excellence in education. 1993. *Journal of Quality and Participation* 16, no. 1 (January): 88–108.

Waesche, J. F. 1987. *Crowning the gravelly hill: A history of the Roland Park–Guilford–Homeland district*. Baltimore: Maclay.

Wainwright, M. 1990. *Miracle cure: The story of antibiotics*. Cambridge, Mass.: Blackwell.

Wajcman, J. 1991. *Feminism confronts technology*. University Park: Pennsylvania State University Press.

Walters, B. R. 1992. Tired of feeling tired? *Amtrak Express* 12, no. 1 (January): 18–21.

———. 1993. Stretching as exercise. *Amtrak Express* 13, no. 3 (May): 18–19.

Walton, M. 1986. *The Deming management method*. New York: Putnam.

Ward, R. 1985. *Red Baker*. New York: Dial.

Ware, N. C. 1992. Suffering and the social construction of illness: The delegitimation of illness experience in chronic fatigue syndrome. *Medical Anthropological Quarterly* 6, no. 4:347–61.

Watts, M. J. 1992. Space for everything (a commentary). *Cultural Anthropology* 7, no. 1 (February): 115–29.

Wells, H. G. [1898] 1986. *The war of the worlds*. New York: Penguin.

Wells, H. G., J. S. Huxley, and G. P. Wells. 1939. *The science of life*. New York: Garden City Publishing Co.

West, N. P. 1992. Young city black men: 56% in trouble. *Baltimore Sun*, 1 September, 1, 13.

White House water samples sent to lab for tests: Research of causes of autoimmune-system disorders of the president, Barbara Bush, and their dog, Millie; vice presidential residence's water tested, too. 1991. *Los Angeles Times*, 1 June, 21.

Whittingham-Barnes, D. 1993. Is there life after unemployment? Yes — if you're willing to stay flexible, acquire new skills and take some risks. *Black Enterprise* 23, no. 7 (February): 180–87.

Why does the body allow foetuses to live? 1985. *Economist*, 21 September, 89.

Wittgenstein, L. 1953. *Philosophical Investigations*. Translated by G. E. M. Anscombe. Oxford: Blackwell.

———. 1967. *Zettel*. Berkeley: University of California Press.

Wolin, S. S. 1989. *The presence of the past: Essays on the state and the constitution*. Baltimore: Johns Hopkins University Press.

Wood, C. 1988. The cold character. *Psychology Today*, April, 13.

Wood, S. 1989. The transformation of work? In *The transformation of work?* ed. S. Wood. London: Unwin Hyman.

Wren, C. S. 1991. South Africa adds spears to township arms ban. *New York Times*, 23 May, 8.

Wren, D. A. 1979. The origin of industrial psychology and sociology. In *Classics of personnel management*, ed. T. H. Patten. Oak Park, Ill.: Moore.

Young, R. M. 1985. Darwinism "is" social. In *The Darwinian heritage*, ed. D. Kohn. Princeton, N.J.: Princeton University Press.

You're not just goldbricking if you have yuppie flu, CDC says. 1991. *Baltimore Sun*, 8 October, 1, 4.

Zukin, S. 1991a. The hollow center: U.S. cities in the global era. In *America at century's end*, ed. A. Wolfe. Berkeley and Los Angeles: University of California Press.

———. 1991b. *Landscapes of power: From Detroit to Disney World*. Berkeley and Los Angeles: University of California Press.

INDEX